THINK
LIKE A
RUNNER

Understanding Why We Run
and How to Do It Better

Jeff Horowitz
Author of *Quick Strength for Runners*

an imprint of Ulysses Press
PO Box 3440
Berkeley, CA 94703
www.velopress.com

VeloPress is the leading publisher of books on sports for passionate and dedicated athletes around the world. Focused on cycling, triathlon, running, swimming, nutrition/diet, and more, VeloPress books help you achieve your goals and reach the top of your game.

ISBN: 978-1-64604-711-6
Library of Congress Control Number: 2024934571

Printed in the United States
10 9 8 7 6 5 4 3 2 1

Acquisitions editor: Kierra Sondereker
Managing editor: Claire Chun
Copy editor: Mary Calvez
Proofreader: Beret Olsen
Front cover design: what!design @ whatweb.com
Interior design and layout: Winnie Liu
Artwork: front cover © SKT Studio/shutterstock.com; chapter shoe graphics © pvgraphics/shutterstock.com; page 114 © Michal Sanca/shutterstock.com

Note: This book has been written and published strictly for informational purposes, and in no way should be used as a substitute for consultation with health care professionals. You should not consider educational material herein to be the practice of medicine or to replace consultation with a physician or other medical practitioner. The author and publisher are providing you with information in this work so that you can have the knowledge and can choose, at your own risk, to act on that knowledge. The author and publisher also urge all readers to be aware of their health status and to consult health care professionals before beginning any health program.

As always, to Stephanie and Alex

CONTENTS

PREFACE

Years ago I found myself sitting on a panel of nine running experts. We were tasked with giving a short talk to a small group on running. I didn't expect a big crowd, but the event proved to be popular; every seat was quickly taken, and people lined the walls and hung about the doorway.

The format was informal. All of the panelists were seated on a dais, where each of us would talk a few minutes about a running topic of our choice and then answer any questions from the audience. My fellow panelists included exercise physiologists, researchers, and doctors.

I had none of those credentials. I had simply parlayed a love of running marathons into a career as a coach, trainer, and author. I considered myself very knowledgeable about running, but I was not an expert on a level with the people on that stage. Given the firepower of the assembled speakers, I was still trying to figure out what I could possibly add to the conversation when the session began. I was seated on the far end of the panel, so I would speak last, for which I was thankful. At least I would get a bit more time to come up with something.

One by one, my fellow panelists began to speak. They talked about biomechanics and fueling, proper foot-strike, and the root causes of running injuries. They talked about the way the body adapts to the stimulus of running and how that could be managed to improve performance.

It was all fascinating, and the audience listened attentively, peppering them with questions. I was familiar with much of this material, but their collective knowledge clearly exceeded my own. As the discussion moved closer to me, I realized that I had nothing meaningful to add to what each of them had said. As the speaker immediately next to me finished his remarks, I felt the first tremors of flop sweat. Then, suddenly, I knew what I wanted to say.

"All of these speakers are clearly experts on running," I began. "They've given us a lot to think about. They've explained much of the science of running, but one thing that hasn't been discussed yet is *why* we run. When we're past mile 22 of the marathon and looking down the barrel of four more miserable miles to the finish line, it's not the science that keeps us going; it's something more. Each runner has to think about why he or she runs and how they can push on when every instinct is telling them to stop. More than biomechanics, it's this willpower that makes us runners."

The nodding heads told me that I had connected with the audience. After the discussion ended, several people came up to me to share their thoughts about the topic I had raised. I realized that as fascinating as it is to hear about the science of running, the most interesting and perhaps challenging thing is to understand what goes on in our heads while we run.

Over the past three decades, I've raced in more than 200 marathons and ultramarathons in every state in the US and all across the globe, from Africa to Antarctica. That's given me a lot of time to think about what I do and why I do it.

I've realized that this topic isn't linear; the questions don't organize in a straight line, like a flow chart. Rather, they spill out in all directions, like children on a playground. Then, as we age, the ground shifts, and all the questions demand new answers. Like life itself.

So let's sit down and discuss this in as straightforward a manner as we can: the mental journey of running. Let's talk about why we began running, how we keep running and manage to fit it into our lives, why and how we race, how we deal with injuries and setbacks, and finally, how we deal with aging as runners. After all, understanding why we run is the only thing that will get us to where we want to go.

CHAPTER ONE

FIRST STEPS

No one has to teach us to run. It's in our DNA, the same way that fish know how to swim and birds know how to fly. Somewhere between 18 and 24 months after being born, after we have mastered walking, we take off at a trot. As Bruce Springsteen sang, "We were born to run."

But *being* a runner, that's a different story. To define ourselves by our running, to identify running not just as something we can do, but as part of who we *are*, is another thing entirely.

I witnessed firsthand my friend Paula's transition into thinking of herself as a runner. Paula was the director of a nonprofit organization that provided services and support to cancer patients and survivors. Part of their funding came from their charity running teams, which were made up of people who had committed to solicit donations in support of their racing goal. As a certified running coach, I designed and oversaw the training program.

One year, Paula decided that she needed not just to support the team emotionally, but to actually join as a participant herself. To put her running shoes where her mouth was, so to speak.

Paula was fit, but she had never run a race before—her sport of choice was golf. But she took her commitment seriously. She dutifully showed up for every weekend group run and did all of her assigned weekday workouts. Entering the second half of the program, she was right on track with her training, but she still harbored doubts.

"I'm not a runner," she insisted during one Sunday workout.

"Paula," I said to her patiently, "we're now in the middle of a 14-mile run. You've been training for months, and soon you're going to complete a marathon." I smiled. "I don't know how else to tell you this, but I think you're a runner."

It would take time—and crossing a marathon finish line—but Paula finally got to the point where she could call herself an honest-to-goodness runner.

That's not an unusual journey for runners. Part of being human is to spend time—perhaps a lifetime—defining who we are. We start as someone's child, and perhaps sibling, then become a member of many things—a school, a town, a team, a religion, a political party, a workplace, a family. Each one of these memberships contributes to how we see ourselves: as committed, loyal, dependable, hardworking, independent, or simply present.

This is how we find our place in the world. We are social animals, and we are programmed to identify with a group, using our definitions of self to locate other folks who seem similar. It's been that way since our distant ancestors looked around the cave and thought, "These are my people."

So what, then, does it mean to be a runner? What did Paula think it meant?

Clearly, it meant more than just being able to run, or to run occasionally. If it's a matter of workouts, how many runs a week do you need before you get your runner's merit badge? Two? Three?

How about racing? Can you be a real runner without racing? What if you run every day but never enter a competition? What if you only train for one race a year, and then don't run after that until the race comes around again?

For me, it was the shoes. I began running, as so many people do, in an effort to shed some extra pounds that had crept onto me when I wasn't looking. I started with some jogging around the block. After doing that for a few weeks, I ran down the street and back. Soon, I was developing routes all across town. But still, I didn't feel like I was truly a runner.

I decided that perhaps my basketball shoes weren't the best footwear for my new hobby. If I was going to continue running, I thought that I should have proper running shoes. So I went to a sporting goods store and gazed up at their wall of specialized footwear. They were all expensive and looked very different from what I was wearing. I tried on a moderately priced pair, found that they felt fine, and bought them. All the way home I wondered if I had just wasted my money.

I needn't have worried. My shiny new shoes felt so much better than my old shoes while I was running. The cushioning and support made my old shoes feel like they were made of concrete, while these new ones softened my every step and seemed to propel me forward. They made me *feel* like a runner.

And there it was. That's when I became a runner. Hundreds of races would follow, and thousands of miles would be covered, but at that moment, heading home with my new running shoes, I had crossed the Rubicon.

For others, it's when they actually cross a finish line. As a coach, I've been lucky enough to work with many gifted athletes. These were people who had already achieved success with their racing, and who came to me for help in reaching their more ambitious goals. It was a joy to train them, but I always felt that my favorite group of runners were the people in my charity groups, like Paula, who had never really run before. The gifted athletes already knew who they were, and working with me would not change that. But when I helped new runners achieve their goals, I knew that I had helped them change their lives.

For many of the new runners, the decisive moment came when they crossed the finish line in their target race. Despite having successfully completed our training program, I could see on their faces that they were still skeptical about being able to finish a marathon. They seemed to think that on race day they would be revealed as frauds, as people masquerading as actual runners. Many of them seemed to believe this through all 26.2 miles of the race.

And then the magical moment happened: They crossed the finish line. The realization of what they had accomplished, of who they now had become, hit them like a thunderbolt. Relief, exhaustion, and elation rolled over them in waves. Many of them sobbed. As a coach, it was my favorite moment, and as I hugged them at the finish line and admired the medals they had just been given, I felt honored to be a part of it.

None of my charity runners ever won a marathon. None of them even came close. But that was never the point. The absolute best part of the sport of running is that there is no minimum standard, no rule, no litmus test that tells you when you are or are not a runner. It is a sport that welcomes you wherever you are and allows you to participate as much or as little as you'd like. Want to walk a bit? Sure. Go off by yourself for a while? Of course. Wear a goofy costume? Knock yourself out. In the House of Running, all are welcome.

You are a runner when you decide that you are a runner.

DO MUDDY RUNS AND GIMMICK RACES COUNT?

You've probably seen them. They're the races that involve more than just running. They've got fierce names and require participants to leap or crawl around, over, under, or through various obstacles. Sometimes barbed wire is involved, sometimes fire, and almost always copious amounts of mud. At the finish line, the only thing visible through the dirt, grime, and yes, occasionally blood, are eyes.

Or sometimes they're just weird. Consider Zombie runs, where volunteers randomly jump out of hiding on a racecourse to chase "regular" participants, and Rainbow runs, where volunteers throw handfuls of colored dust at racers, leaving them a splotchy mess.

It's all in good fun, but are these really races? Is this really running?

To answer this question for myself, I entered a few of these races. It turns out that yes, they were challenging. And I got very dirty. And I had a lot of fun.

These events were timed, and awards were given to the top finishers. I gave it my all in these races, as I imagine many other competitors did, too, and I was happy to see the finish line.

So I guess yes, I have to admit that these are real races, and they can involve real running.

But since I ran those races, I haven't felt tempted to go back and run them again. If a marathon is like a Shakespearean tragedy, giving us new insights with each new viewing, these races are like a rom-com. Fun to watch once, maybe, but not worth buying.

For those who were not committed runners beforehand, I doubt that participating in these events will lead to a lifetime of running and fitness. Regular weekday runs don't involve leaping off docks or scaling walls, and if that's what it took to get you motivated, then putting on your shoes for a 6 a.m. easy run on dark, quiet streets is unlikely to appeal to you.

My advice? Forget the gimmick runs and discover running on your own. Don't just run; *become* a runner.

BECOMING A RUNNER

Let's break this down. For every lifelong habit, there is a first time. For running, where does the decision to start come from?

For many people, the journey began like it did for me: a realization that they need to do more to take care of their health. But there are many, many options available to improve fitness. Why run? I can offer several reasons.

Low entry cost. Running doesn't require membership in a gym or an investment in expensive equipment. All we need is a pair of running shoes, and some people would argue that even those are optional. Even the entry fees for races, which have been going up in recent years, are still relatively low compared with the cumulative price of golf greens fees and ski lift passes.

Low skill requirement. I never took tennis lessons and probably never will. Part of me regrets that because my friends who play tennis seem to really enjoy it. But not knowing how to play—even a little bit—keeps me from trying it. If I were to take up tennis, I know that it would require a commitment to starting from scratch with a teacher and spending many long hours practicing before I could rise just to the level of mere competency.

Running, as we've said, is nothing like that. There's a surprisingly large amount to learn to be a good runner—more on that later—but there is very little that needs to be learned right at the start. In fact, there's no simpler sport in the world: You simply need to run from here to there. If it's a training run, just do it comfortably. If it's a race, try to do it as fast as you can. And that's it; the whole world of running in a nutshell.

Low embarrassment risk. Most of us are nervous when we try something new, often because we worry about looking bad while doing it. We fear that other people will see us, leaving us feeling foolish or perhaps even humiliated.

This is not a baseless fear. If you're lining up at the golf tee and preparing for your drive, it's hard to ignore that the rest of your foursome has their eyes on you, as does the foursome waiting patiently behind them. It occurs to you that it is very possible that, despite the golf pro's advice from your last lesson, you'll pull your head up as you swing, which will result in another topped ball. You can see it as if it already happened: the ball falls off the tee and rolls just a few feet as the seven other golfers look down and sadly shake their heads.

There's no equivalent to that scene in running. Embarrassing things can and do happen—all runners have at least one, if not many, embarrassing potty stories—but for the most part, there's not a lot that could go wrong that would leave you feeling embarrassed or humiliated. Anyway, most runners are paying too much attention to their own training and racing to spend energy jeering anyone else.

Strong positive reinforcement. Almost every run provides its own incentive to run again. Even runs that feel difficult in the beginning usually end with the runner glad for having gotten out the door and feeling good about what was achieved.

There are several reasons for this. First, no one—*no one*—feels great right from the start. The human body is a machine that needs to warm up before it runs well, and that takes time. Joints have to become lubricated, muscles need to get warm and become pliable, and the heart has to start pumping blood faster. It can take anywhere from a few minutes to the better part of a half hour or more for all this to take place. Experienced runners know this. Don't judge how you feel in the first few minutes; it's always possible for a seemingly bad run to turn good. Let the old jalopy get rolling before you decide what kind of day it is. Once it gets going, things can get better very quickly.

Second, we must remember that genetically, our bodies have not moved far from the jungle, where the law of the land was eat or be eaten. When running to catch prey or to avoid becoming prey, there was no time to worry about a sore knee or tired legs. Your body evolved to deliver adrenaline to give you a quick burst of energy and to mute discomfort, and that system still works today, even when you're dodging poodles and parked cars instead of lions.

Third, running is a great antidepressant. Research has shown how helpful running is as a mood elevator, in part because your body will give you plenty of endorphins and other happy chemicals to make running a fun experience. This is true not just for people with diagnosed clinical depression, but for all of us. Whenever I feel my optimism and enthusiasm slipping, I know that a run with help bring me up again.

Years ago, when I was in my first year of law school, a fellow student told me that she had been having trouble dealing with the stress of upcoming exams, and she went to see her doctor. He prescribed antianxiety medication for her. Now, I'm not a doctor, but without a diagnosis of clinical depression, wouldn't it make sense for her to start with a run or walk outside before taking medications?

Fourth, running provides a great space for meditation and problem solving. Running allows your brain to enter into a meditative space where free-form thinking is possible. When your conscious mind is not being forced to engage deeply, the subconscious mind is free to roam and explore. When the brain is so engaged in the present moment that it loses track of time, a kind of mindfulness results. This has come to be known as the "flow state," where concentrating on a specific task helps the brain minimize distractions and maximize productivity and performance.[1]

This is a highly creative space, where brainstorming and problem solving most easily take place. I've known runners who carry notepads to jot down thoughts, or who record messages to themselves on their phones. Whether it's coming up with a solution for a work problem or figuring out how to deal with a delicate family issue, the best ideas all seem to come up while running.

High success rate for races. Running is not a zero-sum game, like tennis or softball. No one has to lose for you to win. Sure, someone has to come in first in a race, and maybe your loud-mouth neighbor will beat you and never let you forget about it, but the perfect race is still one in which every person who starts the race finishes it. I always pose this question to my new runners: Do you know what they call the person who comes in last in a race? A *finisher*. And keep in mind also that even if you come in last in a race, you are ahead of all the

---

1 The flow state was first identified by Mihaly Csikszentmihalyi, whose groundbreaking work triggered a tidal wave of research. While based on scientific observation, this research has become part of our accepted cultural knowledge, as athletes at all levels talk about the thrilling moments of being "in the zone," when their bodies seemed to perform at a high level without requiring conscious thought. See, generally, Mike Oppland, "8 Traits of Flow According to Mihaly Csikszentmihalyi," www. PositivePsychology.com, December 16, 2016.

THINK LIKE A **RUNNER**

hundreds and thousands of people who didn't even try. Don't think that you need to run a long race, either, if you decide to give racing a try. There's a distance for everyone, from a "fun run" mile, to a 5K, to an ultramarathon, and lots in between. They are all true race experiences.

I recall a 5K race that I once ran with my son, who was a young toddler at the time. I ran with a baby jogger, and he would try running for a little while, then climb into the stroller to take a break while I pushed us along the course. The race route was a figure eight, with the start and end points right in the middle.

After completing the first loop to the right, my son and I passed the finish line on our way to completing the second loop to the left. My son saw the finish line and realized that we were passing it. He drew the only logical conclusion: "This race is never going to end!" he yelled out in alarm.

Just then, my son heard the race announcer remind the runners to grab a banana after crossing the finish line. He grew quiet as he processed this new information. "Everyone gets a banana?" he asked me uncertainly. I nodded. "Bananas for everyone!" he called out triumphantly.

And there you have it: the entire race experience in two sentences. "It feels like it will never end. But it will, and then there's food."

The runners around us smiled and laughed because they could appreciate the way in which even a toddler was able to grasp the essence of our sport.

WHAT ABOUT YOUR FRIENDS?

Like any joyous discovery, you will probably want to share your new passion for running. After all, after you explain how wonderful it is, won't they want to join in the fun?

Not necessarily. This is an area in which you want to tread lightly. People come to running for many different reasons, and they often stay away for just as many varied reasons. Maybe it just doesn't feel good to them, or maybe they're intimidated by it. Maybe the runs that you find peaceful and invigorating are just boring to them. Or maybe they take your encouragement to be a criticism of their current lifestyle. Whatever the reason, don't be surprised if you find that the more you urge someone to run, the more they push back.

A better approach would be to lead by example. Once they see how much running has added to your life—by making you healthier and happier—they might start asking you questions about getting started. They might even ask if they could come with you on a run sometime.

This is the moment for you to be an ambassador for our sport. Take them for an easy run and answer all the questions—the ones they've asked *and* the ones they should have asked. But don't get out too far in front with your encouragement; you may turn around and find that they've stopped following you. But if you limit yourself to being available and supportive when they bring up running, they will come to it at their own pace.

Or they might not. In fact, they might look at you as someone who has joined a cult, and a potentially dangerous one at that. This is especially true if they find that you will no longer join them for some of the old activities that you used to enjoy together—like going out drinking and eating late into the night—because you have a long run scheduled the next day. They may tell you that you've changed, and that you're no fun anymore.

Are they right? To some degree, they probably are. You *have* changed; that's the point. But be sure that you haven't picked up some bad habits along with your good ones. Be an ambassador, but don't be an evangelist or preacher. Make sure that you still give your close friends—including your non-running friends—time and attention. Friendships, like plants, wither in darkness. Don't let that happen.

Continue to give your friends time and attention, and in all likelihood, they'll come around. They might never fully understand the role that running plays in your life, but they will probably come to accept it. They may even cheer you on at races, and take you out to brunch afterward. After all, they are your friends, and once they see that running makes you happy, they'll accept the new you.

You might find, however, that for a small number of friends, accepting your new love for running is a bridge too far, and there might not be anything you can do to change that. You might have an argument over this at some point, or you may just drift apart.

It might sound unfeeling to say this, but not every person you meet can be a forever friend. But cheer up! Through running you will meet a world of new people who share your passion and understand your priorities.

When I was new to running and had just been bitten by the marathon bug, a friend of mine predicted that if I kept up with my long distance running habit, my bones would eventually turn to dust. That was many years ago, and from all indications, I'm no worse for the wear and tear of decades of running and racing. I've had my share of injuries, but all of these problems eventually resolved, leaving me free to continue to run, usually pain-free. Running is still a part of my life. Unfortunately, that friend isn't.

Membership in the tribe. To be a runner is to belong to a group. There are no membership cards or secret handshakes, but when runners pass each other on the roads and trails, they usually nod to each other or raise a hand slightly in greeting. They might never have met before, but nevertheless they feel that they know each other.

That's because running itself generally indicates a certain set of values—a belief in the value of hard work and of persevering though discomfort, maybe even pain. All runners have learned patience and how to appreciate the natural world in which we are just a small part. Perhaps most important, they know that anyone can have a good day or a bad day, that the distance between the two is shorter than you might think, and that everyone does better with a bit of encouragement.

This is the creed of the running tribe. The tribe doesn't care what your body size or shape is, how fast you are, or how many races you've run or plan to run. You can talk with other people in the tribe, make plans to run with them, become lifelong friends with them, or only give that little nod in passing. The tribe doesn't care. The only requirement to be a member of this tribe is that you run. For many people, this makes it the best group in the world.

These are the logical reasons for running. But for many of us, there's something deeper, something that's harder to express, something almost spiritual about our connection to running. We experience the world through running in a way that no other activity allows, in a way that leaves us transformed.

With no effort at all, I can conjure up a dozen incredible memories that I've experienced as a runner. Being the first one out on a snowy morning and turning around to see my solo footprints trailing behind as far as the eye could see. Hearing the cracking of the river ice as winter loosened its grip during a February training run. Crossing a bridge during a driving rainstorm, feeling more like I was swimming than running, but also feeling more alive than I ever had before. Running in a pack in the Comrades Marathon in South Africa when the runners around me spontaneously began to sing the beautiful work song "Shosholoza," a song of hope that had become the country's unofficial national anthem. Seeing dozens of heartbreakingly beautiful sunrises and tiny purple flowers by a wood trail's edge. All to the steady rhythm of my footsteps.

I come back from every run feeling like I am a better person than when I stepped out of my house. I feel more at peace and more determined to be a better husband, father, and friend.

What could possibly top that?

But none of this happened without taking that first step out the door. Deciding to get out and run is different from actually doing it, and sports psychologists have recognized that there are several distinct steps involved in moving from planning a lifestyle change, to actually making it happen.

The first step is *contemplation*, where you consider the change, like imagining what it would be like to get out and run.

The next step is *planning*, where you identify the specific steps you would need to take to get running, like buying running clothes.

Next comes *preparation*, where you take specific steps to begin running, like marking your calendar, setting your alarm, and laying out your clothes.

Finally comes *execution*, where you get out and run.

MAKING IT STICK

It all looks quite straightforward, but sometimes it isn't. Someone might take the first two steps toward becoming a runner, and then get distracted or discouraged and need to start over. Or they take all the steps, and then get sidetracked, only to realize some time later that they had unintentionally quit.

The most successful people recognize that berating yourself for past failures is never productive, and that no matter how many false starts there are, the next one could be the one that sticks. There is no deadline or three-strikes rule in running, so take as many turns as you need to get onboard. The trick is to figure out what kept the plan from working in the past, and to make the necessary changes to find success the next time. Here are some typical deal-breakers many beginning runners face and some suggestions for overcoming them.

NOT ENOUGH HOURS IN THE DAY

This is the big one. Running takes time, and for many people, free time is something they just don't have, and that's not going to change. But that's OK. You can still be a runner. With some planning, you can make it work.

If you don't have much time, don't waste time. Lay out your running outfit the night before so that you don't have to look for things in the morning. You can even wear those clothes to bed and save that step in the morning.

Do a little personal time management assessment so that you can see where you waste time. You might find that you get sucked into chat-rooms, online videos, and social media. To paraphrase the counterculture mavens of the 1960s: turn off and tune out.

If you can't do the run you want, want the run you have. You may not have an hour to run, but do you have thirty minutes? With exercise, it is vastly better to do even a little bit than none at all. Do what you can, and you'll be better for it.

Or do you have twenty minutes now and twenty minutes later? The positive physiological effects of running are cumulative, so a couple of short runs add up. And psychologically, even a short run can leave you feeling productive and energized.

SAFETY CONCERNS

I wish that this were an irrational fear, but there have been too many reports of runners being attacked to ignore the threat. It's a relatively rare event, but there are ways to make it even less likely.

Run with friends. The old saying is true for runners: there's safety in numbers. Coordinate with a friend, join a local running club, or see if your neighborhood running store hosts group workouts.

Run only on busy well-lit streets at night. Street crime often happens in the shadows, so try to avoid them. If you can't find any nearby roads that are safe to run on, consider driving to a safer road, or even taking your workout indoors to a treadmill.

Take a self-defense class and carry a loud whistle. This won't guarantee your safety, but it might give you enough of an edge to come out on top if something should happen that you couldn't avoid. At the very least, this will increase your sense of control and raise your self-confidence.

Run with a dog. A dog will love you unconditionally and protect you to the death. How many people in your life can you say that about? Still, I understand that this isn't an option for everyone. Perhaps your landlord has a rule against having pets, or maybe you job involves working late hours and traveling. Not a problem. If your neighbor has a dog, offer to take it for a little run. Both the dog and your neighbor will be thrilled with your offer.

FEELING SELF-CONSCIOUS WHILE RUNNING

This is another problem that could be solved by running with a dog. People will assume that you're just trying to give the dog some exercise, and not the other way around. If you don't have a dog, offer to take your neighbor's dog for a run.

BOREDOM

People often assume that because running is such a big part of my life, I must love every minute of it. That's just not true. Running is by its very nature repetitive. The joy comes from the moments—and these don't happen all the time—when you feel strong and fast and almost immortal. The rest of the time it's a matter of just putting one foot in front of the other. But there are some strategies that you can deploy to inject a little fun back in your workouts.

Change your route. Running down a different street, or on a different trail, or even just running in the opposite direction on your usual loop route can make a tired routine seem fresh.

Catch up with a friend. Instead of getting coffee or lunch with an old pal, see if they'd be willing to connect for a workout and chat. Obviously, this is dependent on your friend being a runner also, but as you make friends in the running community, this should become a more feasible option.

Problem-solve. The best time to try to figure out solutions for your work, homelife, and other personal issues is while running. That's because, as we talked about earlier, running can create an almost meditative state, which is ideal for creative thinking and brainstorming. Answers to sticky questions, which had eluded you earlier, may suddenly flash brilliantly in your mind during a run. Before you realize it, you will have finished your run.

Be patient and have faith. Boredom often comes when you focus on how difficult running feels, and when you keep wishing for the ordeal to be over. As you get more fit, running won't feel so difficult, so your mind can wander instead of reminding you how miserable you are.

This switch can even happen during the course of a single run. As you warm up during the beginning of your run, a lot of changes are taking place, as we discussed earlier. Your joints get lubricated with synovial fluid, your muscles get warm and pliable, and your heart rate increases to deliver more oxygen and nutrients to your muscles. All this will make you feel better, so don't judge your run by how you feel in the first few minutes— or even the first half hour. That could change.

I'm reminded now of a marathon I once ran in Jamaica. It was a double out-and-back course, which meant that we had to run out in one direction, turn around and run back, and then run past the start line in the other direction, and run back to the finish, where we had originally started.

I felt miserable during the entire first out-and-back of the race. I was sluggish and tired and distracted and not enjoying any of it. This went on for nearly two hours. I even considered dropping out as I went past the starting line.

But then something changed. I suddenly started to feel better. It was like I had just woken up. My breathing settled down, my stride began to quicken, and I began to pass people. Running suddenly became fun.

What had seemed earlier like a terrible mistake had become one of my best races. If I had quit earlier, I never would have discovered that wonderful new place that my body was about to glide into.

The lesson that I learned is that endurance running is a sport of redemption. There is always time to turn a bad run around, and a sublime moment might be just minutes away. Have a little faith.

Get distracted. This is not always the best strategy—and we'll talk more about that later—but sometimes it's the one we need. If you're running on a treadmill, which, as all runners know, is where fun goes to die, set up a screen to watch your favorite mindless action movie or comedy. Don't pick anything too serious or complicated; it's often hard to focus intently on anything while running.

If you're running outside, listen to music or an interesting podcast. But don't forget the need to be safe. Stay aware of your surroundings, and don't keep the volume so loud that you can't hear what's going on around you. The new bone transducer headphones allow you to listen to your device without blocking the ear canal, so you can have your cake and eat it too while running, so to speak.

YOU KNOW YOU'RE A RUNNER

Are you still unsure about whether you're a runner? There's no single set definition for a runner, but there are many, many indicators. If you find yourself agreeing with at least 10 of the definitions listed below, you can consider yourself a runner.

- You own more running shoes than dress shoes, and the running shoes are more expensive.
- You plan vacations around races.
- Your knowledge of the metric system is limited to 5K and 10K.
- You know where to find working fountains and available public bathrooms anywhere in your city.
- You wake up earlier for your weekend run than you do for work.
- You know what a PR and a BQ are.
- You have no problem discussing poop and pee with your friends.
- The first thing you do when visiting a new place is to scope out running routes.
- You know what a fartlek is, what pronation is, and what VO_2 max is.
- When someone says "Thanksgiving," you think "Turkey Trot."
- Your partner insists that you leave your running shoes outside the door.
- You have more old race numbers than family photos.
- You've been accused of treating food as fuel.
- You think a shower should be earned.
- You think cool and cloudy is perfect weather.

- You consider running to be a viable commuting option.

WHAT TO THINK ABOUT WHEN YOU RUN

This is a big topic, and the subject of one of my most frequently asked questions. Distance running doesn't require the intense focus that other sports require. If you are a cyclist and you lose your concentration while you're in a race, you can crash and cause serious injury to yourself and those around you. But if you lose your focus on a run, you're just someone walking down the street or in a park. So without the threat of bodily harm to worry about, what should you think about to keep your brain busy?

We briefly touched on this when we talked about combatting boredom, but there's more to be said here. As you develop as a runner, you'll find that you need to train your mind as much as your body. In time, and with practice, you will be able to quiet your thoughts and settle into a calm state that you can sustain not just for minutes, but for hours.

This won't happen overnight. In the beginning, it will occur to you during a long run that you still have miles—and maybe hours—to go before you're done, and your mind might scream with anxiety and frustration. Treat it just like you would a screaming child, with soothing words and distracting messages. Try to focus on something else, anything else, instead of what you are doing.

Over time, you will find that not only can you get through these long runs, but that you treasure them. This is your private time, when you can be attentive to your own needs and no one else's. If most of your professional and private day is spent, like mine, in conversation with other people, running can be a time to take a well-earned break from talking and listening; it can become a time for rejuvenation.

But that's not the end of the story. To become better runners, we need to take a deeper dive into the question of what to do with our brain while running; we need to explore the difference between dissociative and associative thinking.

DISSOCIATIVE THINKING

Dissociative thinking occurs when you try to distance yourself from what you're experiencing by introducing distractions. This is what you're doing when you listen to music or a podcast while running. Consciously or not, you're trying to think about anything other than how hard it is to run so that the minutes will fly by and you'll be done before you know it.

Dissociative running can also be the necessary choice if there's something on your mind that requires your attention. Maybe you'll need to make a difficult phone call later that day or you need to process something that happened that's upset you. Thinking this through while running may be the best way to handle your problem.

Dissociative running can also be the right approach on days where you're feeling less motivated and you just want to get through your run. My tagline for such runs is "It may not be pretty, but I'll get it done." Being distracted is often the only way that I can make that happen.

ASSOCIATIVE THINKING

Associative thinking, on the other hand, occurs when you keep focused on your running instead of trying to ignore it. This kind of focused thinking can be further divided into being internally or externally associative.

Internally associative thinking focuses on how you're feeling. Imagine that you have a checklist of questions that you run through every time you run: Are you too cold or too hot? Are you hungry or thirsty? Tired? Is anything hurting? You can also use this as an opportunity to check on your form. Are you hunched over or slapping your feet? Are you remembering to swing your arms instead of rotating your body? These are all examples of internally focused thinking.

Externally associative thinking focuses on what's around you. Perhaps there's a broken sidewalk up ahead or a hill looming in front of you. Or maybe you see storm clouds rolling in. These are all conditions that will require your externally focused attention.

If you are interested in improving your running performance, as well as running safely and reducing your risk of injury, associative thinking is the necessary approach. Internally associative thinking gives you an opportunity to address any bodily issues that you may be having, to the extent that you can. If you are thirsty or hungry, it might be time to take a nutrition break. If you need a restroom, now would be the time to make a beeline to a nearby café or store. If you are tired, you can slow down or cut the workout short. If something hurts, perhaps you need to stop running and check in with your doctor. If your form is falling apart simply because you're tired, you can refocus on correcting it. In all these events, paying attention to what you're feeling will help you make the run productive and keep you from making a possible problem worse.

Externally associative thinking helps you respond to your environment and adjust your mindset or form to deal with any imminent challenges or problems. Trail runners are especially adept at this, since every step requires a quick assessment of the risk of tripping over roots and rocks. Similarly, if you live in a northern clime, you have to always be on the alert for black ice and other slippery conditions during the winter. If you see bad weather developing during your run, or have any other concerns about your safety, you may even need to abandon your run altogether and seek shelter or help. Externally associative running will also warn you about any potential threats that you might encounter on your run.

Which of these approaches you choose depends on what your goals are for that run and the conditions that you find yourself in. If you are training for a race and hoping to do well—and more on this in a later chapter—then you'll need to be associative. Most competitive runners train and race this way. But if you are running primarily to stay in shape and take a break from life, dissociative running can be the way to go. This is especially true if you are running on a treadmill, where you won't have to worry about road conditions, bad weather, or (usually) safety.

Keep in mind that this is not an either/or situation. You can shift from one mode of thinking during the course of a season, a training cycle, or even a workout. Go with what feels right in the moment.

GEARING UP

As I described to you earlier, the process of buying my first pair of running shoes is what transformed me into feeling like an actual runner. This can be true not just for shoes, but also for all running clothing and gear. When you buy running clothes and shoes, you are making a commitment. Sure, there are many people who buy running shoes not because they plan to run, but just because they are comfortable, but that's not the case for you; you're buying them for a specific purpose, and this is no small investment. When you spend the money, you are giving yourself a big incentive to use your new gear as you intended. After all, no one likes to waste money.

Let's get this out of the way now—do not feel guilty for what you are about to spend on running gear. You are making an investment in yourself, and you deserve it. Even with this expense, running is a cheaper sport than many others. If you doubt me, talk to your skiing or golfing friends. I love cycling, and I love my road bike, but for what I spent on that bike I could have bought twenty pairs of expensive running shoes.

Also, you are now a runner, and runners wear technical clothes for a reason: *they work*. Cheap cotton is a bad choice for running shirts and shorts because when they get wet, they stay wet, which makes you colder when it's cold out, and hotter when it's hot. Technical non-cotton clothing wicks sweat away from your body and dries quickly, which keeps you more comfortable. This is true even down to your feet: cotton socks cause friction between layers of skin in your feet, which leads to painful blisters. Avoid cotton to avoid problems.

Good running shoes in particular are worth it. They can help correct certain flaws you may have in your feet and in your form, and they will give you a stable platform for all that follows. You deserve to share in these benefits, so don't skimp.

Running gear also tends to be long lasting. Your shoes will probably need to be replaced before your clothing does, but even so, they should be good for 300 to 500 miles or more, depending on your form and usage. So if you suffer a case of sticker shock when buying shoes, take a deep breath and figure out the expected cost per mile. You'll find it easier to reach for your credit card.

We *need* good running gear. But buying and using running-specific clothing isn't just about their engineered performance-improving qualities; it's about creating the psychological environment for success in running. When I change into my running clothes, I am removing myself from my sedentary lifestyle and transforming into something else, something faster and stronger. It's almost a heroic act, like a knight putting on armor, or like Superman slipping into his costume. I am preparing myself for battle.

To be most effective, in my experience, you must believe that your clothing *looks* fast. I once had a pair of bright, neon-peach running shoes. They demanded so much attention that even I noticed them while running, as they flashed in and out of my peripheral vision. Once, when I showed up for a workout wearing them, a friend of mine said, "Anyone wearing shoes like that had better be fast." Looking down at my shoes, I felt certain that I *would* be fast. Like Dorothy's ruby red slippers, I felt that my running shoes had power of their own, and that by wearing them, I could tap into that power.

This is an example of the placebo effect. In the classic example, a person is given a dose of medicine and is told that they should soon feel an improvement in their condition. And then they do, even though the "medication" they were given hasn't been shown to have any therapeutic value.

The reason these fake pills work is because the person expects them to work. When they are told that the pills will help, this becomes a self-fulfilling prophecy. The body responds to the belief that the medicine is real and will work, and the person reports that their pain is reduced. Or in the case of wearing fast-looking running shoes, the person performs with greater effort in training or racing. Another term for this phenomenon is *confirmation bias*, which is where the brain believes something is true because we were told that it's true. So we expected it to be true, and our bodies responded to it like it was true.

The fascinating thing about the placebo effect is that studies are now starting to show that this occurs even when the patient knows that the treatment is fake. Something about merely thinking about the medicine—real or not—creates an involuntary positive response in the body.

What this means for us is that, if you believe that a red shirt or new shoes will instantly make you a faster runner, it's possible that they will, even if you know in your heart that this is an irrational belief. So buy the best-looking clothing and shoes that you can, in the color option that you feel best about.

WHAT GEAR YOU'LL NEED AND WHERE TO GET IT

Below is a short list of running essentials. Whenever you see the word "Technical," simply think "non-cotton."

- Technical lightweight T-shirt or sports top
- Technical running shorts
- Tights
- Gloves
- Knitted hat
- Cap
- Socks
- Technical long-sleeve top
- Lightweight running jacket
- Running shoes

The best place to buy these items is a neighborhood running store. Not only will you be supporting the establishment that probably contributes so much to your local running community through sponsoring races and holding free weekend group runs, but it's also a place that will offer you expert advice on what gear and products might fit your specific needs. They might even have a treadmill set up so you can check your form and they can match you with the corresponding shoes that will work best for you. These shops also stand behind their products, and are often willing to exchange shoes or other items after miles of use if it turns out that they are not working out for you.

Beyond your local store, there are many quality online sites that offer good prices. But in order to shop these sites, you really need to know what you're looking for because there will not be an expert available to walk you through it.

Further down the list is your local discount clothing chain. These stores offer the lowest level of service, but the best prices. Running clothing is usually mixed into their athletic wear or active wear departments. If you have the time and inclination to pick through the racks, you can sometimes find great name-brand running clothing at a fraction of the retail price.

Also, most big-time races have expos associated with their packet pick-up. This is a good place to check out the latest and greatest new products, as well as pick up older products at bargain prices.

WHAT IF RUNNING REALLY ISN'T WORKING OUT FOR ME?

A runner should like to run. Not all the time, but often, and most of their runs should feel good.

If this isn't true, despite the wonderful clothing you're wearing, the great route you've chosen, the friends you're running with, or the music you're listening to, perhaps it's time for you to reconsider your relationship to running. Ask yourself what, if anything, you enjoy about running. If you are always trying to ignore what you're doing when you run, if running *never* seems to bring you any joy, maybe you should be trying something else that you actually like.

I've known people who hate to run but run anyway because they know that it's a good way to stay fit. That seems very sad to me. Life is too short to spend time doing things you don't like, especially when there are other options. Try riding a bicycle, swimming, or hiking. And do so without guilt.

But before you turn your back on running, give it a fair shot. I've known people who quit running because they never believed that they really could do it. That's not a fair basis for quitting because I know for a fact that almost everyone can run. Some people will inevitably run faster or farther than others, but everyone runs.

If, on the other hand, you can do it but you don't *want* to, then that's fine with me. You simply don't like running. After all, there are many things that I know I *could* do, but that I won't ever *want* to do. Bungee jumping, for one. That sport has zero appeal for me. You might think it's the closest you'll ever come to touching the face of God, but I still don't want anything to do with it.

Here's a thought experiment: What are the activities in your life in which you lose track of time? What are you doing when you look up at the clock and suddenly notice that a few hours have flown by? These are the activities that you love. If any of them involve regular, steady movement, that's the exercise for you, and that's what you should be doing more often.

It comes down to this: an important axiom in personal training is that the best exercise is the one that you'll do. I'm lucky in that I enjoy running. I love it on a physical, emotional, and intellectual level. I have been lucky enough to be in a position to share that love with other people, many of whom find that running leaves them feeling the same way. But after giving it an honest effort, if you find that running isn't for you, then go and find the thing that is.

CONGRATULATIONS— YOU'RE A RUNNER!

If you've gotten this far, you have made the leap to a big change in your lifestyle. You have redefined who you are—no small feat!—and you now probably look at the world, and your place in it, in a different way than you did before. You are a runner, and you are now connected to a worldwide community.

If you doubt the truth of that last statement, let me tell you a story. I once was helping a friend organize a charity race in Addis Ababa, Ethiopia, to benefit an orphanage for children of AIDS victims. The driving force behind the race was a former Ethiopian businessman who had moved to the United States many years before, but who still maintained very close ties with his homeland. He hoped to put on a race not only to raise money for the orphanage but also to raise awareness of its important work. Through mutual contacts, he was put in touch with me to help him turn his vision into a reality.

I had some experience in race management and working with nonprofits. I was moved by what he told me of his mission, and I took on this project as a volunteer. Some months later, after a lot of groundwork, I found myself in Addis Ababa, doing preparatory on-site work for the upcoming race.

Addis is the largest city in Ethiopia. It is the capital of the country and also a political center of Africa since it's home to the African Union and many embassies. Still, Addis seemed far different from my home in Washington, DC.

I wanted to get in some running while I was there, but I wasn't sure where I could go. I was told that there was a nearby outdoor amphitheater that locals used for their workouts, so early one morning, I set out at an easy jog to find it.

As I made my way to the training ground, I came across another runner heading in the same direction. We silently fell into step together, aware that we apparently had the same destination in mind. When we arrived, I saw dozens of runners sprinting up and down the concrete steps of the outdoor arena. My companion and I looked at each other and began doing the same.

We worked hard, in complete silence, and at the end of our workout, we turned to each other and smiled again. I was wearing a pair of running sunglasses—nice, and of moderate value, but just one of several similar pairs I had back at home. Seeing that my companion had none, I took off my sunglasses and held them out to him. He accepted my gift graciously. We smiled at each other once last time, more warmly now, it seemed to me, and then we left the arena and went our separate ways.

My training partner and I had not uttered a single word to each other, but we were runners, so we didn't need to. We knew all that we needed to know about each other at that moment, and we were able to share a meaningful experience through our mutual love of running.

Running will do that for you if you are open to it. It will bring the world to you and connect you to people everywhere through your shared passion. But only if you want it to, and if you take the time and trouble to seek it out.

Being a runner also means that you have to figure out how to settle into this new lifestyle and make it fit into all the other parts of your life. It's like moving into a new house and seeing all the unopened boxes and plastic-wrapped furniture stacked in your new living room: you know it will all work out, but you're still going to have to work hard to figure out where everything goes.

In the next chapter we will take a look at this process, figuring out how to manage your running for the long haul.

CH-CH-CH-CHANGES

After you've been running regularly for a few months, you will no doubt become aware of how much better you feel. You don't get winded anymore when climbing steps, you sleep better, and you feel like you've got more energy. None of this comes as a surprise to you; you had read about the changes that come from running, and you were expecting them. But do you really know what's going on under the hood? The details are just as fascinating as the results. Here's a look at what's going on in your body:

- **Increased mitochondrial density.** You may remember from biology class that mitochondria are the powerhouses of the cell. They are the structures in the cell where energy is produced. An increase in the energy demands of the body, as induced by running, leads the body to make more mitochondria, which increases your available energy level.

- **Increased fuel storage.** As you demand more endurance from your body, your body responds by increasing the amount of glycogen it stores within its muscle cells. This fuel is readily accessible and will enable you to run farther and faster.

- **Increased utilization of stored fat.** Fat is not your body's favorite fuel source, but it is calorically denser than carbs, so it is more efficiently stored than glycogen. Even the thinnest marathoner has enough stored fat to help fuel a strong race. As you push your body to endure longer and longer runs, your body begins to access these fat stores more readily, delaying the point at which you run out of fuel.

- **Stronger muscles, tendons, and bones.** The body reacts to the stress of exertion and impact by improving its ability to handle these loads. It does so by resculpting itself—making the muscles stronger, the bones denser, and the tendons tougher.

- **Improved capillary network.** Through a process called neovascularization, the body responds to exercise by broadening its capillary network, which increases its ability to deliver oxygen and fuel to working muscles and to remove waste products.

CHAPTER TWO

TRAINING

You're now a runner. You've learned the ropes and have made running a regular part of your life. At this point, you've got some new choices to make.

First, you have to decide what you want from your running. What are your goals? Let's spend a little bit of time talking about how we can answer this question.

SETTING RUNNING GOALS

I once brought my friend Dave to a gym as my guest, and rather than breezing through, as we anticipated, he was stopped by the sales team for a chat before he was allowed to hit the workout floor. As an icebreaker, the salesperson asked Dave about his fitness goals. Dave, annoyed by the delay, looked at the salesman and deadpanned, "I have no fitness goals." That pretty much ended the conversation.

That actually wasn't true for Dave, and it shouldn't be true for you. Now that running is a significant part of your life, you should be able to articulate what it gives to you and what you hope to get from it in the future. But there are many reasons to run and many goals that you might have for your running, so it can be difficult to figure out what role running plays in your life.

I believe it's worthwhile to give this some thought. If you can articulate your reasons for running, you can decide if your goals are realistic and if your actions are bringing you closer to meeting your goals. This is the essence of being *purposeful*. To get you started on thinking about your goals, let's review the list of reasons that often motivate people to keep running.

LOSING WEIGHT

This is a big one. In fact, it was my initial goal when I started running regularly. Running is often the first go-to option that people think of to shed excess fat, and it makes sense. Running is a big calorie burner—in general, it takes 100 calories to run a mile,[2] so a daily five-mile run can eat up 500 calories a day. A pound of fat holds approximately 3500 calories, so if you run five miles a day for a week, you can shed a pound of fat per week. That can add up to over 50 pounds a year. That's a pretty big return on your time and energy investment.

But there's a problem here. Running should not be your primary tool for weight loss. Fitness trainers have a phrase to

---

2 This can be a little confusing, and the numbers can vary a bit depending on a person's weight, but as a general rule of thumb, this is a good, simple equation to rely on. Note that this is much different than calculating calories burned *per minute* of running. If you looked at it that way, running fast burns more calories than running slowly, but that doesn't contradict our 100 calories per mile rule because a fast runner would simply be getting in more miles in the same amount of time spent by a slow runner. But my best advice: don't overthink this.

describe this dilemma: you can no sooner train your way thin than you can eat your way fit. What this phrase means is that it's best to think of improving fitness and losing weight as related but separate goals.

Here's why: training works by introducing an exercise stimulus, which triggers an adaptation response. In other words, when you push your body a bit more than it's used to, it responds by improving. Your body adds muscular strength and cardiovascular conditioning in order to meet the new demands that you have placed on it. This, to me, is the magical part of training: you ask your body to improve by working a little harder, and your body does so.

But there's a limit to this process. If your stimulus is greater than your body's ability to adapt, you can get hurt. We've all fallen into that hole. We run too far, too fast, too soon in our training program, or we lift too much weight in the gym, perhaps sacrificing form. The next thing we know, we've got a nagging ache.

Or perhaps we just refuse to take a day off when we should. A key part of training is to give our bodies a chance to respond to a stimulus by resting. When we take down time—particularly when we sleep—our bodies release human growth hormone, which triggers the repair and improvement of our muscles and tissue after exercise. If you don't rest, your body won't have a chance to repair itself. Your body won't improve, and an injury is likely right around the corner.

Now consider how this process might conflict with your weight loss goals. We had said earlier that you could lose about a pound a week by running five miles every day. But suppose that after six days of running, you're feeling tired and sore. The sensible thing would be to take a day off and let your body rest before you resume your routine. But if you are committed to burning 500 calories a day, you may decide that you have to ignore your body's warning signs and push through another workout to hit your calorie-burning goal.

You may get away with this for a while; perhaps your soreness will simply pass. But it's more likely that the soreness will develop into a real injury. Then, instead of needing to take just a day off from running, you may be forced to take several weeks off.

Or consider this: I tell my clients that the physical and mental benefits of one really good workout outweigh any benefits from two subpar workouts. This means if I feel sluggish and tired after warming up and starting my routine—past the initial hesitancy that my body usually approaches every workout with and well into the time when I should be feeling energized and enthusiastic about my workout—then I shut the workout down. I've literally stopped running and have turned around and walked home. I'm not happy about doing so—I have to quiet that stubborn part of my brain that yells at me to keep going—but I know that if I rest now, I will almost certainly have a much better workout tomorrow.

Another reason you should not rely on running alone to lose unwanted body weight is that it's far too easy to overestimate the calorie-burn of running and underestimate the calories consumed during eating. If, as we've said, you burn about 100 calories for every mile you run, and you've completed that 5-mile daily run you've committed to, then you've burned about 500 calories. You should feel good about that. You might feel so good that you decide that you can treat yourself to a nice lunch that you were craving all during your run: a cheeseburger with fries. That doesn't sound like an unreasonable reward for exercising for almost an hour, so you head to your favorite diner.

But that little meal packs in 800 to 1,000 calories, which is almost double what you've burned by running. If this becomes your regular habit, then instead of losing a pound of fat every week by running, you will *gain* a pound every week.

The better approach to pursuing a goal of losing weight, then, is not to rely just on running, but to focus as well on your food choices. If you eat a healthy diet and exercise regularly, you will almost certainly hit your goals.[3]

Think of exercise and healthy eating as being two friends that support each other. They enjoy their time together and help each other out, but they have their own separate lives and needs. Similarly, good eating will fuel good workouts, and good workouts will improve your body's food absorption and calorie burn, but your workout plan and your eating plan should be on separate, if parallel, tracks.

A final word about having weight loss as a goal: while the health benefits of being at an appropriate body weight are well established, including a lowered risk of diabetes, many types of cancer, and cardiovascular disease, this can be a fraught area for

---

3 I am not a certified nutritionist, and this is not the place to talk about the details of a good eating plan, but I love the simplicity of advice given by nutrition author Michael Pollard, set out in his book *In Defense of Food* (Penguin Books, 2009): "Eat food. Not too much. Mostly plants. That, more or less, is the short answer to the supposedly complicated and confusing question of what we humans should eat in order to be maximally healthy." There's a lot to be said about proper nutrition, and I encourage you to talk with a nutritionist if you have any questions, but following these three rules would be a great place to start.

many people because of misconceptions about what it means to be healthy. In our thinness-obsessed culture, many people confuse being lean with being fit, and view any excess body fat with the same disdain that they treat dog poop on the sidewalk. This is not only a wrong viewpoint, but it's also potentially dangerous.

Research has shown that it's better to be moderately overweight and active than to be thin and sedentary. That is to say, movement is more important than thinness. If you regularly exercise, you will be at a lower risk for illness and early death, regardless of your weight. Of course, it's best to be active and also be at an appropriate body weight, and obesity carries a wide range of health risks, but my point is that you should not obsess about your body shape. Just get out and move, and you will feel better. Chances are that you will look better, too.

GET HEALTHIER

This is a great goal for runners. The health benefits of running are many and well documented. They include the obvious ones, like improved cardiovascular health and weight management, but there are many others as well, some of which are surprising. Researchers have documented that running improves your digestion, the quality of your sleep, your sexual function, and even your hearing. Basically, running makes everything better.

It also doesn't take a lot of running to achieve these benefits. The key is consistency; if you run regularly, you will be healthier. You don't need to go very far or very fast, although there are benefits to doing that as well. The latest recommendation from the American Heart Association is that to maintain good health, we should all get at least 150 minutes of moderate aerobic exercise per week, or 75 minutes of vigorous activity. [4] That's an average of just 30 minutes of easy running 5 days per week, or just two or three hard runs of 20 to 25 minutes. That's only a tiny fraction of the time most of us spend mindlessly looking at social media every week.

It gets even better: the benefits of exercise are cumulative, which means that your daily workout doesn't even have to be done all at once. You can run 15 minutes in the morning and 15 minutes at night, and you'll hit your goal. If you are able to work this into your daily routine, perhaps by incorporating it into your commute, or while running errands or taking your dog for a walk, then you won't even have to set aside any additional time to hit your fitness goals.

That is, unless you want to. Many runners—and I count myself among these—think of our runs as sacred time. We use our runs to focus on ourselves, to recharge our emotional batteries, to have a quiet moment, and to escape the stress that most days bring. It's our refuge, and we are very protective of it. If our goals are moderate, which they usually are, as most training runs are an hour or less, it's not hard to fit into the day. It can be squeezed in before breakfast, or during lunchtime, or perhaps right before dinner. One way or the other, we can make it work.

Eventually, most of your friends and family will respect your need for this time alone. They will see that you are more even-tempered and happier after running, and they will come to support your need to lace up your running shoes.

---

4 See heart.org/en/healthy-living/fitness/fitness-basics/aha-recs-for-physical-activity-in-adults.

Or perhaps, instead of being a refuge, running becomes your social time. You can coordinate with friends to run together, and your daily or weekend runs become a regular appointment that strengthens bonds of friendship. Humans are social animals, and you may find, as many of us have, that time spent running with friends is the highlight of your day. I've shared stories, worked through problems, laughed, and sometimes just given silent support to my friends while running.

The goal here is to use running—whether done alone or with friends—to add balance to your life. Once again, the goal is consistency, rather than quality. You don't have to be fast, you don't have to suffer; all you need to do is get out there as often as you can every week.

GET FASTER

This is a goal that sometimes sneaks up on runners. You begin running to shed a few pounds, and then you settle into a routine where you meet friends for a run or go out for an invigorating run by yourself, and you are happy.

But then a race suddenly falls into your lap. Perhaps a friend is doing a 5K to support a charity and asks you to join them, or you read about a Thanksgiving Turkey Trot in the neighborhood, and you're intrigued. You sign up for the race, line up at the starting line, the gun goes off, and you surge forward with the pack. You run harder than you ever have before, and you gasp as you cross the finish line. You are exhausted, but elated. You look at your watch, and you've run faster than you ever have before. Your breathing quiets down, but your feeling of accomplishment lasts all day. You are so pleased with yourself. Then a strange thought enters you mind: Could I run even faster?

That's the hook. Now you've discovered racing. You don't have to abandon your easy or social runs, but your world has just expanded into something more serious. Running faster takes effort—more training, planning, and, yes, suffering. But it will be worth it because that feeling of elation that you felt during your first race will be there for you with every finish line. Or, at least, it could be. And that's what pulls you in to training with serious intent.

Making the jump from casual runner to competitive runner is a shift in goals. While competitive running should be a healthy pursuit—and, for most of us, it is—it requires a different mindset than casual running. The stimulus on your body will be greater, but so will the risk of injury. Balancing training load with recovery is a major challenge for competitive runners at all levels. But even the most sophisticated and complicated training plans begin with a simple and clear understanding of the difference between result goals and process goals.

RESULT GOALS

Result goals are the big dreams that we hope to achieve. In running, this can be getting an Olympic medal, winning a race, qualifying for the Boston Marathon, or simply completing an event. These are the goals that motivate us to get out of bed in the morning and struggle through difficult workouts. We push on because we have that brass ring in our sights, and we want to reach up and grab it, so much so that we are willing to endure months (even years!) of hard work to get there.

The problem with these goals is that they are simply too big, and there are too many things outside of our control that could derail us. A result goal can capture the imagination—in fact, it is probably the only thing that really does—but it can also feel overwhelming. I've run many marathons, but the idea of running 26.2 miles still, after all these years, seems too immense to wrap my head around. If I think about it too much, I begin to get discouraged.

In addition to the distance, I think about the other factors that may derail my dreams. Suppose I hope to win a race. I will be competing against other runners, but who are those people? I have no say over who will show up or what condition they will be in. Or suppose that it rains or snows on race day. What am I to do about that? The more you think about it, the more you realize that so much of racing, and life, depends on the favorable inclination of factors entirely out of our control.

This is a humbling and sobering thought, but it doesn't need to be a crippling one. As legendary football coach Vince Lombardi said, luck is preparation and opportunity. Get ready, hope for the best, and you may yet achieve your dreams.

PROCESS GOALS

Now *process goals* come into the picture. These are the day-to-day goals that you set for yourself. They are almost completely within your control, and while they may be difficult, they are manageable. Process goals are simply the steps you take on the way to your result goals, the minute-to-minute choices and efforts that you make that end up defining who you are.

A process goal could be as simple as committing to waking up a half hour earlier every day to work out. Your process goals end up including everything about your workout routine: committing to doing a speed-work session every week, to doing your long run every week, to getting more sleep and eating better. Every little decision that you make is a part of your process, and every successful completion of your routine—waking up early, getting out the door, eating healthy—is a process triumph.

The hope and expectation is that if you successfully hit your process goals, you will achieve your result goals. Or, more accurately, you will put yourself in a favorable position to achieve your result goals, as long as the factors out of your control don't block you.

For me, this is the answer to the daunting enormity of running 26.2 miles. Running that far is surely impossible, I tell myself. But after getting through my training program, I know that I can run one mile 26 times in a row. Somehow, that doesn't sound so bad. After all, it's just a matter of putting one foot in front of the other. Process yields results. Simple.

We'll talk more about racing later—that's a subject all its own. Your job now is to use this framework to consider what your own goals should be, keeping in mind that your goals likely will change over time. Whatever goals you choose, you will have to rely on your training program to achieve them. We'll talk about that next.

SUSTAINABLE RUNNING

Consistency and sustainability. These should be the hallmarks of any healthy training program. Our goal should be to create a lifestyle that keeps us healthy and that we find fulfilling. Whether we run for peace of mind or to finish first in our age group, running should be a positive part of our lives.

This sounds obvious, but in practice it's not so simple. I've had many clients who have been strongly committed to doing everything they had to do to get better—everything, that is, except rest. These were people who were dedicated enough to run, but not dedicated enough to *not* run when necessary.

This leads to one of our big, overarching rules. Write this one down in capitals on your bathroom mirror.

Be smarter than you are brave.

As with all our big rules, it is true not just in running but in life. When I introduce this rule to my clients and teams, I have them think on it in silence for a few moments. It is deceptively simple, but, as coach Walt Whitman would have said, it contains multitudes.

To understand the importance of this rule, we have to first accept that we are all strong, determined beings. You would not be a runner if you weren't stubborn. Running requires that you get out of bed when you'd rather not, get out the door on a cold or wet day when you'd rather stay inside, and struggle through a difficult workout when you'd rather quit. You force yourself through all this because you are a devout believer in the value of delayed gratification. You make the deposits in your fitness account every day because you know that it will accumulate and yield incredible interest, to be spent lavishly on race day when you pass your friends on the way to the finish line, or perhaps when you go to your high school reunion and shock everyone with your youthful vigor.

But more than this, being tough has come to define who we are. We are the people who do the difficult things that other ordinary mortals are unable or unwilling to do. We get up early and do the hard workouts, day after day, week after week, because we are just those kinds of people. We are the superheroes in our own movies, and superheroes do not take days off.

Except that superheroes are fictional, and real people need days off sometimes. If you can accept that you are indeed a powerful, motivated, and exceptional person, then you should be able to realize that, having achieved this exalted status, you have nothing left to prove. You can take your imagined reputation out of the equation. In other words, you can start thinking with your brain instead of your ego.

DO NOT OVERRULE YOUR BODY

This will come up in many situations where discretion is the greater part of valor. If your Achilles tendon has been complaining to you, perhaps you need to skip this week's speed-work session. Not because you are weak, but because letting your body heal is the smart thing to do. Or perhaps you need to skip that race, or most difficult of all, drop out of a race after having started.

This is sacrilegious talk among some runners, especially those who would rather die on their shields than give up the battle. But consider this: professional runners—those exalted humans who are so gifted and determined that they could actually earn a living by winning races—drop out of races *all the time.* They do this because they know that their bodies are their greatest assets, along with their minds, and that it is absolutely reckless to batter their bodies pointlessly. If they feel an injury coming on, they will shut down a workout or even a race in order to avoid shutting down an entire season. They listen to their body, and they do not ignore what it tells them.

One of the greatest marathoners of all time, Paula Radcliffe, was the reigning world record holder when she lined up for the start of the marathon at the Athens Olympics in 2004, the favorite to win a gold medal. But Paula had been struggling with a leg injury, and the race did not go as she hoped. She eventually had to drop out late in the race. "I've been back time and again in my mind," she later explained. "I know I was called a quitter a lot at the time and criticized for stopping. I think something in my mind kicked in, in self-preservation. I knew that I wasn't going to be able to finish, that I wasn't going to push my body to complete collapse that day."[5] Paula's wisdom in protecting her body—in being smarter than she was brave—paid off when she won the NYC Marathon that fall and the gold medal in the marathon at the Helsinki World Championships the following year. Those successes would never have happened if she had broken her body in the Olympics earlier.

BE OPPORTUNISTIC

But that's not the end of the story. Being smart about running is not just about holding back and being cautious; it's also about taking chances when your body feels ready to go.

I call this being opportunistic. Like a fledgling bird that is suddenly ready to leave the nest, you will have days when you were planning on doing a limited, low-key workout. But then, for some unexplained reason, you suddenly feel as if your legs are two steel springs ready to unleash their power. On those days, don't hold back—let them run free! Those "Look, Ma, I'm on top of the world!" kinds of days don't come around all that often, so when they do, take advantage of them.

---

5 "Paula Radcliffe on 'the One that Got Away,'" *Athletics Weekly*, August 8, 2020.

Of course, you should still be smart about this and keep your workout within reason. Don't suddenly double your long run distance, or sprint longer and faster than you ever have before. You don't want to end up with an injury. Just be willing to push yourself if your body gives you the green light. Go a little bit farther or a little bit faster than you were planning to. How far and how fast? That's up to you—or, more accurately, your body—but a good guideline is that your effort should still feel relatively moderate.

PARTNERING WITH YOUR BODY

Part of being a purposeful runner is to have goals for every workout. These don't have to be very ambitious or challenging—although they might be—they just have to be the result of conscious choices that you've made based on a thoughtful review of what you and your body need and can handle. When you understand this, you are able to work in partnership with your body.

Partnering with your body means that you will be attentive to its need for recovery and rest after hard efforts and that you will structure your workout routine with this in mind. This doesn't have to be a complicated process, however. Here are four rules of thumb that will set you on the right path.

The Shorter the Run, the Harder the Effort. As a runner, you should have different gears available to you, just as a cyclist or a race car driver would, to enable you to go slower or faster as the circumstances require. You employ these different speeds to satisfy different goals. For example, if you're building your base by doing long runs, you would expect to run slower so as not to put too much stress on your body. By the same token, if you plan to run fast, you would aim for a shorter distance so that you can sustain your target pace.

With this in mind, you can look at your workouts the other way around, focusing on time instead of length, and setting the pace accordingly. If your day's schedule only allows you to do a short workout, you can make up for the lack of time running by raising the intensity. Or, if you have the luxury of having a big block of time, you may decide that you can finally do that long, easy run you've been planning.

Alternate Hard Days with Easier Days. It's unrealistic to think that we can run fast all the time. When we push our bodies through a hard workout, we have to pay the price, which is to allow it to recover from the hard effort. If we fail to do this, and instead push our bodies hard all the time, we court injury. Knowing how this works gives us the opportunity to plan for this ebb and flow by intentionally varying our efforts during the course of our weekly runs.

Take At Least One Day Off Every Week. This is as much for your mind as your body. No one can push endlessly doing anything day after day, week after week, without hitting either an emotional or a physical wall. That's true even for the things you love, like running. Plan to take a day off from running every week. Sleep in, have a nice breakfast, do a crossword puzzle. Enjoy the break. You'll come back stronger from it.

Don't Bully Your Body. These might sound like conflicting suggestions—slow down, except when you should speed up!—but in fact they are just flip sides of the same coin. The common thread that connects our rule to run smart and our rule to run opportunistically is the goal of running in partnership with our body.

It would be helpful here to think of your body not as who you are, but instead as a very close friend. Treat your body with love and respect, and it will give you everything it has to give. Shakespeare wrote in *Julius Caesar*, "Bid me run and I will strive with things impossible," and that's what your body wants to do for you, but you need to work within its limits. Or, as I like to say, don't bully your body.

I understand that to be a long-distance runner is to have a greater capacity for enduring pain and ignoring the body's signals to stop. That's all to the good, but there comes a time when we all need to stop being so willful and stay within the realm of the possible. When your body starts to break down—when soreness gives way to sharp pain that does not go away quickly—it's time to back off your training and let your body rest.

As you get more experienced, you'll be able to interpret what your body is telling you more and more efficiently. Instead of waiting for an ache or pain to appear, you may realize that your sluggishness and lack of enthusiasm are early warning signs of trouble ahead.

You ignore these signals from your body at your peril. Bullying your body into complying with your workout and race goals, despite the negative biofeedback that your body is supplying to you, never ends well. Let's repeat that: *it never ends well*. At best, you'll waste your energy on subpar workouts, which neither advance your fitness nor leave you feeling confident and elated. And at worst, it can lead to an injury and a long layoff.

TAKE YOURSELF SERIOUSLY

This directive is fundamentally about your mindset as a runner. I see too many runners who don't think that they deserve to be treated as real runners. They might not say that in so many words, but their actions speak volumes.

To be a real runner is to seek out and make use of all the possible tools to improve as a runner and to become as good as your desire and talent will allow. This includes having access to the gear and tools that runners use and to the coaching and medical support that help athletes excel. When told of these options, however, many runners turn sheepish and say something like, "Well, I'm not a real runner, not like *that*."

This is a mistake. It's like saying that although you have a driver's license, you don't deserve to have a good car because you're not a professional race car driver.

Don't make that mistake. Everyone improves with training and support. If you've decided that your goal is to improve as a runner, then you deserve to make use of all the tools at your disposal.

You might be thinking right now that cost could be a barrier. I won't minimize this expense, but it might be lower than you think. The purchase of gear is generally a one-time or rare expense, and the use of a supporting team of health-care and coaching professionals can be surprisingly affordable. But in my experience, it's not the actual cost that stops people from making use of these resources. After all, these are some of the same people who don't blink at ordering expensive coffees at their favorite cafés. It's actually the voice in their head that says they are not worth it as runners, that they are not talented enough to justify spending this money.

I'm reminded of a client of mine. She is a good athlete, and she has completed many triathlons and marathons. But she is not an elite athlete. She has never finished in the top three of any race, or, as elite athletes like to say, "podiumed." Still, she hired me as a coach and trainer. She told me that when she mentioned this to a friend of hers, the friend was very surprised. She explained to her friend that coaching is not just for Olympic hopefuls; anyone can get a coach. It had never occurred to her that somehow she wasn't good enough to get coached. In fact, she understood that it was quite the opposite: she hired a coach because she felt that she could get better, and she knew that a coach could help her reach that goal.

Let me be clear: if you run, you absolutely deserve to have the best support that the community can offer you. This is not a frivolous expenditure or a rare treat. This is an investment in your health, and it will actually save you money and aggravation down the road. Consider it on par with your regular doctor or dentist visits; spending money on the gear and services that will help you run will reduce the money spent on medical care and physical therapy you will incur down the road if you get injured.

What follows is a list of services and equipment that I believe you should have access to in order to stay healthy and to improve as a runner. None of them are absolutely essential; there are great runners who have never used any of these resources. But I believe that all of these can help you, sometimes dramatically so. Look through the list and decide for yourself. Talk to your running friends and check in with chat rooms to discuss these options. You might be surprised at how many people will tell you that using these resources was worth every penny to them.

GAIT ANALYSIS

This is an important investment in yourself, and it surprises me how few runners have it done. Think of it like a home inspection: you only need to do it once, or perhaps every few years, but the knowledge you gain from it will be a blueprint for what you need to do to save yourself time and money down the road.

A gait analysis is essentially a review of your running form by a trained professional who knows what they're looking for. They will see what kind of runner you are, and explain it to you in layman's terms.

For example, there is the mythical perfect runner, the person who has perfect foot-strike and body position and movement patterns, who glides over the road like they're filled with helium, barely touching the ground, barely breaking a sweat. Gait analysis would only confirm their perfection and feed their confidence.

And then there's the rest of us. We all try to run as best we can, despite our flat feet, high arches, poor core strength, and bad form. I often think back to a shirt that I once saw a runner wearing during a race. It read, "I'm not hurt; I just run like this."

But it doesn't have to be this way. We can fix problems with our form and stride, and become better runners, but only if we know what exactly we're doing wrong. That's where a gait analysis comes in.

First, you need to find a trained professional. As a certified and experienced coach, I am adept at spotting many problems with form, and I provide that service for my clients, but I am not qualified to do a full analysis. Neither is the salesperson at your favorite shoe store who offers to watch you run down the street or on the store treadmill. We are all well-meaning, and can offer some good advice, but you deserve and need more.

Find the physical therapy clinics in your area and ask if they do gait analysis. You can even check in with your local university to see if their department of exercise physiology offers gait analysis. These establishments have staff that are trained to do a detailed clinical analysis—far more in-depth and reliable than what a coach or shoe salesperson can provide.

Here's how it will work: They will put you on a treadmill and film your running. Then they'll review it in slow motion in order to show you what they have seen. They will probably email you the footage so you can review it later at home. Next, they will explain what flaws you have in your running form—and yes, in all likelihood, there will be flaws. Targeted exercises and drills can correct some of these. Others may require you to buy specific shoes or orthotics. But these problems can be corrected, and your therapist will explain how.

Then it is up to you to go home and implement what you were told. This may not be fun; as runners, we really just want to get out and run, and anything else is a distraction or an annoyance. But remember: you went through the trouble of paying for a gait analysis in order to run better and stay healthy. Be smart and make it happen.

MASSAGE

Having regular massage is, at least to me, one of those things that I used to think was only for the rich and famous. Not so. Therapeutic massage helps restore proper range of motion and muscle function by breaking up adhesions in the muscle tissue. These are the clusters of fibers, also called knots, that can result from hard use. Think of muscle fibers as a bowl of spaghetti. Instead of being in perfect alignment, these fibers can get tangled and stick to one another. Deep-tissue massage breaks up these adhesions and helps move waste products out of the muscle tissue, which promotes healing and recovery and results in greater range of movement.

If you use your body regularly and ask it to perform great tasks like running for hours, then you owe it to your body to treat it well in return. Not just once, but often. Again, think of your body as a car. You know that you need to change your car's oil and get tune-ups to keep it running well. Not just once, but regularly. Your body is no different. The benefits of massage don't all accrue after just one or two sessions; your body requires regular maintenance.

Some years ago I was dealing with soreness in my upper back, just to the inside of my shoulder blades. This is a common spot for pain, since the muscles of this area—specifically, the rhomboids—work hard to keep you upright, especially when you are bent over a computer screen. On top of that, there is a nerve cluster in this area, and it is here that stress often accumulates and manifests as soreness and pain.

I was getting regular massage at the time to deal with this issue, as well as to generally work through soreness throughout my body that was the result of my training. During one particular massage session, I was lying on my stomach as the therapist probed deeply into my rear shoulders and upper back. Suddenly, I was completely drenched in sweat. If you've ever experienced flop sweat right before public speaking, or broken out in a cold sweat when your plane hits bad turbulence during a flight, this experience was like that, but much, much worse. I was soaked, and so were the towels on me and under me.

I was embarrassed (maybe mortified is closer to the truth). I felt that I had to address the elephant in the room, so I muttered some kind of apology to the therapist. He was unsurprised and unconcerned. "This happens all the time," he said. "When your body suddenly lets go of stress, it can be very dramatic." It had taken weeks of work to get there, but apparently my rhomboids and surrounding muscle had finally relaxed.

So, how often should *you* get massage? That might be a better question for your financial adviser than your coach, because if it were up to me, I would recommend getting a massage every day. In my fantasies of a perfect life, that's what I would have. I've never read or heard of any instance where someone suffered for having too many massages. But like many people, I don't have the time or money for that. Instead, I recommend having a massage at least once per month, or every few weeks if you're dealing with a specific issue, like a tender Achilles tendon, a sore back, or a hamstring issue.

FOAM ROLLER

Similar to massage, foam rolling helps maintain good muscle tone, range of motion, and function. But unlike massage, foam rolling can be done by yourself, and it only requires a one-time purchase of a relatively inexpensive piece of equipment.

Foam rolling used to be the province only of physical therapists, but it has now moved out into the popular culture. Foam rollers can be easily found in most sporting goods stores and online. You'll find many options: short travel rollers, knobbed rollers, and even electric rollers that vibrate when you use them. I recommend getting a full-sized plain roller—it will be about 36 inches long, made of moderately dense foam.

Foam rolling involves the massage of your muscles, but it also affects your fascia. Fascia is the connective tissue that is found throughout your body. Like kitchen wrap, it holds things in place and provides support. Think about the film you saw covering raw chicken parts the last time you were preparing that for dinner. That's fascia.

Fascia serves an important function in the body, but fascia can also get tight and inflamed. If you've ever had the common runner's injury plantar fasciitis, you know that's an inflammation of your fascia on the arch of your foot.

Foam rolling helps reduce tightness in fascia throughout the body, reducing soreness and inflammation. For that reason, foam rolling is technically known as *self-myofascial release*.

Using a foam roller is relatively simple. There are many online classes and tutorials that can help you learn the basics of foam rolling, but essentially it works like this: you use your own body weight to press down on the roller while you roll back and forth, providing a massage to the targeted area.

So, for example, if you want to work on your hamstrings, sit crosswise on the roller and then move your body back, rolling down along the back of your legs until you get to your knees, and then roll back up again. Similarly, you can roll back and forth on your calves, or flip over and roll out your quadriceps muscles on the front of your thighs. You can also position your body to roll over your outer hip, your lower, middle, and upper back, and even your shoulders.

In general, I recommend rolling back and forth over each body part five times. If you feel soreness or discomfort, you should spend a little more time on that area, rolling or even just staying still and pressing down.

You may find that foam rolling can be very uncomfortable, perhaps even painful. When I first began foam rolling, I was quite a sight—I grimaced, yelped, and almost screamed. But over time the muscles relaxed, and now I hardly feel any discomfort at all as I go through my foam rolling routine. In fact, I use my foam roller to help me find any soreness that I might be unaware of and need to address with rest or further massage.

As with massage, the benefits of foam rolling can take weeks and even months to manifest, but improvement will occur. The key, as with so many endeavors, is consistency. You should aim to foam roll several times a week, and even daily, if possible. It doesn't take long to do—only 5 or 10 minutes per session—

so you should make it part of your daily routine as you would taking a shower or brushing your teeth.

MASSAGE GUN

Electric massage guns are a relatively new tool available to runners and other athletes. They use a percussive hammer to work on soft tissue. Similar to massage and foam rolling, they help loosen knots and reduce stress in muscles and fascia, thereby promoting recovery and healing after hard workouts. I don't consider this tool to be absolutely essential—if in doubt, make sure that you have a foam roller, if nothing else—but I find it to be very useful.

Massage guns vary quite a bit in cost and quality, and I recommend getting a mid-level brand. The highest-priced models don't seem to me to be worth the extra expense, and the very cheapest brands seem noticeably inferior.

As with massage, you can use this mode of self-care as often as you like; a few minutes spent with this daily as you're watching the news or your favorite show is time well spent. I've expanded past targeting the obvious muscles—my quads, hamstrings, and calves— and now try to work on all my reachable soft tissue, including the palms of my hands and the soles of my feet. Does all of that improve my health? I think so, though I can't prove it. But I can tell you this: it feels great, and it makes me happy, and that alone justifies its use.

SEQUENTIAL COMPRESSION SLEEVES

Developed originally for people with circulatory problems, electric sequential compression sleeves are now marketed to endurance athletes. They zipper up over your legs, from your ankles to your hips, and inflate like a blood pressure cuff, squeezing your legs and in the process, in theory, promoting blood flow and forcing waste products out of your legs after a big workout.

The sequential part of this treatment occurs when the separate compartments of the sleeves compress and release in a pattern set by the program you've chosen on the attached monitor. You can work each of the four chambers in order, from the bottom up, or engage groups of them in different patterns. You can also adjust the intensity by regulating the inflation.

As with the massage gun, I consider this tool to be useful but not essential. I recommend that you try it and decide for yourself if it feels productive to you. Personally, I can't say for sure that it has helped my performance or recovery, but as with the massage gun, it feels good, and using it always relaxes me, so it's valuable to me if only for those reasons, especially since the model I have is modestly priced.

COACHING

I'll say up front that I'm biased on this topic since I am a running coach myself. But keep in mind that I don't recommend hiring a running coach just because I am one; I *became* a running coach because I saw the value they bring to runners, including myself.

Coaches provide structure and direction to a running routine. They create detailed training programs containing daily workouts, direct individual workouts, and help athletes set and attain performance goals. They also provide racing strategies and, following the key event, post-race analysis.

But a coach provides much more than all that. A good running coach is also a collaborator, a cheerleader, and a confidant. A coach provides support for the one area in which so many runners, even accomplished elite athletes, are deficient: confidence.

A coach can convince a doubting athlete that they can, in fact, achieve their dreams, and they do so because they have the credibility that comes from instructing and training athletes every step of the way. When a coach tells an athlete that they are ready for a peak performance, it's not just wishful thinking; they have objectively viewed the athlete with an expert's eye, and they know what is possible, even if the athlete has doubts.

The best coaching arrangements work as partnerships. The coach brings their expertise and judgment, while the athlete brings their knowledge of their own body and what kind of training works best for them. Together, a good coach and an experienced, self-aware athlete can develop and prod the athlete to perform up to his or her potential.

As you may gather from this discussion, the best use of a coach is in pursuit of a specific goal. In general, I work with two kinds of athletes in my own coaching practice. The first are runners who are just starting out and, literally, want to set out on the right foot. These runners know that having expert advice is always the best way to start out.

The second are athletes who have a defined racing goal, whether to complete a first marathon, attain a Boston Marathon qualifying time, or even aim for an Olympic Trial berth. For all of these athletes, working with a coach provides invaluable guidance and support. The question is not whether they deserve coaching; the question is whether they think they could use the help in attaining their goals. For many of them, the answer is yes.

Most run coaching, then, is a specific tool designed to address a specific challenge. Think of it as you would your expensive winter coat: when you need it, you *really* need it, but when you don't, you can put it away.

In other words, if you're starting out and you want expert advice, or if you decide that you want to take on a racing challenge, then coaching can be a great tool for you to use. For the rest of the time—perhaps the greater part of your entire running life—you can happily and effectively be your own coach and confidant.

But there is still another way in which coaching can be useful to a runner, even one who is not working toward achieving a performance goal in an upcoming race. In these other cases, coaching provides *accountability*.

Knowing that a coach is waiting for you for a workout and will be watching you is a powerful incentive for many people to show up, especially if they've paid good money for the service. It's also a commonly observed phenomenon that all athletes, including me, work harder and perform better when they are watched. Maybe it harks back to our childhood, when we wanted to show off for our parents in the playground and yelled out, "Look what I can do!" For whatever reason, I know I dig a little deeper and run a little harder when a coach has their eyes on me. Can we put a price on that kind of motivation? For many runners, the answer is yes, the coaching fee, and it's worth it.

Where to Find a Coach

If and when you decide that you would like to work with a running coach, there are several good places to find one.

Local Running Store. More than just a place where you can buy gear and shoes, running stores have become more like community centers for local runners. Many offer coaching for group workouts, and often the staff can give recommendations and contact information for individual coaching.

Physical Therapy Clinic. These offices often have good working relationships with local coaches because coaches want reliable therapists for their injured athletes, and clinics want to be able to refer healthy athletes to coaches they trust. So check in with local clinics for coach recommendations.

Local Gym. Many gyms have certified running coaches on their staff, and if not, can often recommend coaches in the community. The coaching and personal trainer community in most areas is relatively small, and practitioners can usually recommend specialists they know personally.

Running Clubs. Similar to running stores, many local running clubs offer professionally coached workouts to their members, often at no cost above the club membership fee. Members and officers of the club are usually familiar with coaches in the area and can offer recommendations for coaches who can be contacted for one-on-one workouts.

Road Runners Club of America. The RRCA is an umbrella organization for running clubs large and small across the country. Its main purpose is to share information and best practices to its member clubs, as well as to offer insurance for club races. It also offers a coaching certification program and maintains a database of its certified coaches. You can find RRCA-certified coaches in your area by checking their website: https://www.rrca.org/coaches.[6]

Your Running Friends. Perhaps the best resource for finding a good running coach is your local running community. Ask around and seek out recommendations from your friends who have had a positive experience with a coach, and then interview the coach yourself.

---

6 Full disclosure: I am an RRCA Level II certified coach myself.

Choosing the Best Coach for You

When you interview your prospective coach, ask about their education. Do they have a degree in exercise physiology, or are they certified by one or more nationally recognized organizations (such as the RRCA, mentioned just above)? Ask about their experience, both in running and coaching. Ask also for references, and follow up by interviewing these athletes with whom they've worked.

Finally, and perhaps most importantly, ask your prospective coach about their coaching philosophy. Even after you've established a coach's qualifications, you want to know that they are the kind of person you can work with.

I've read that there are two kinds of coaches: the fine detail coaches and the big block coaches. The fine detail coaches try to address every possible aspect of training and racing, under the theory that if you can control as many factors as possible that go into making a good race, then your chances for success will be greater. These coaches obsess on details, making them a good fit for runners who likewise want to control as many aspects of their lives as possible in order to feel confident and secure.

Big block coaches, on the other hand, try to make sure that the most important elements of training are covered, without worrying about the smaller details. They trust that as long as their clients have done the important work in training, they are positioned for success. This kind of coach works for runners who are not great at getting all of the details in their lives in order, and who are comfortable with a little bit of life's natural chaos. They know from experience that most things seem to work out and don't like to worry about every bad thing that could happen but probably won't.

Neither the detail coach nor the big block coach has the perfect approach; success is a matter of matching the coaching style to the athlete. As with many of these types of definitions, most coaches are probably a little bit of both. Keep this in mind as you talk with your prospective coach. And trust your instincts. We all base our feelings on things that we're consciously aware of, as well as many things that we don't even know that we know. My wife, for example, is a great judge of character. I have absolutely no idea what she bases her opinion on, and I'm not even sure that she does, but over the years her gut instincts have almost invariably proven to be right.

Remember, you can always change coaches and approaches if something isn't working for you. You should never feel like you are permanently locked into an arrangement. After all, the coach is working for you, not the other way around.

But I would ask you this: once you choose a coach, give that person a chance to implement their program before you evaluate it. Sometimes the benefits of a coach's approach are not immediately available, and the seeds of excellence that they plant early need time before they blossom. Or fail. But if you've committed to using a coach, give the process a little time before you judge the results. How long? Perhaps a season, or at least a few months. That's up to you.

Hopefully, by this point, you have committed to taking yourself and your running seriously. You are a regular runner who knows what to do to take care of your body and how to get the support you need to maintain and improve your running.

I'll leave it to you to devise your training plan; there are plenty of guidebooks out there to help with that task, including my own. Our job here is to develop the mindset to continue to run, regardless of the training plan you're working under. With that in mind, we'll now turn to different topics in training that often present obstacles to runners. Our goal is to overcome these roadblocks and keep moving forward.

CAN TWO BE BETTER THAN ONE?

I hear it often: "I don't always have time to do my long cardio workout all at once. Can I just do two short workouts in the same day?"

The quick answer is a qualified yes, as we briefly discussed earlier. If your main goal is to burn fat, then two-a-day workouts are fine. Exercise is cumulative, so everything you do counts—your quick 15-minute elliptical warm-up in the morning, the stairs you climb during the day, your lunchtime walk, and your after-work 30 minute treadmill run all add up to burn fat and get you in shape.

If your goal is to prepare for a race, it's a little more complicated.

Our bodies store about two and a half hours' worth of glycogen, or blood sugar, and when that's used up, like late in a marathon, we "bonk" or "hit the wall." It takes several days to fully replace lost glycogen, but when we train our bodies to burn fat along with the glycogen, we can stretch out our glycogen supply. Since fat is more than twice as calorie-dense as sugar, even a little can go a long way. When we do long workouts, we are training our bodies to do just that and avoid hitting the wall.

Here's the interesting part: since it takes several days to restock glycogen, all aerobic activity done on the same day—in any increments—will encourage fat burning because our bodies won't have new sugar to turn to. So a two-a-day routine encourages fat burning just as much as a single long workout.

Further, if your goal is to get faster in your sport—say, running or cycling—you might find that you can do each of the two shorter workouts at a faster pace than the single long workout because you've had a little rest in between them. Extra bonus!

But if you are preparing for a race, remember that unless you're doing a relay, most races are not split up in segments. So, for example, if you line up for a marathon having never run more than 10 miles in a row at one time, then you will be entering into uncharted territory. That's not what you want on race day.

There's also the risk of burnout. Running two-a-day workouts can often feel like one workout too many.

The bottom line: use two-a-day workouts when your schedule demands, or to shake up your training, but try not to rely too heavily on them.

RUNNING THROUGH THE SEASONS

For many runners, especially those who live in the north, one of the joys of running is experiencing the changing of the seasons up close and personal. However, during the course of the year, these runners may have to accommodate a swing in temperature of 100 degrees or more. Much of this can be exciting and beautiful to witness, but it can also present many challenges.

Within that wide range, there's a sweet spot where the temperature seems ideal for running. Runners have debated what this ideal temperature is since, well, for as long as there have been runners. The consensus seems to be that the best temperature in which to run is in the upper 40s to low 50s Fahrenheit.

That's not me. As all of my friends, family, clients, and students know—really, almost anyone who has ever talked to me—I hate being cold. Hate it.

This isn't something new. When I was a child of maybe five or six, I remember stepping outside on a summer day. I remember being hit with a gust of heat, like I had just stepped into a furnace. But instead of being uncomfortable, I took a deep breath and enjoyed the moment. It felt to me like my grandmother was hugging me in a loving embrace.

That's warmth to me.

Cold weather, on the other hand, is hateful. When you step out the door on a cold day, there's just a moment when you are still protected by a little bubble of warm air that you've brought with you from indoors. But the cold quickly pierces that bubble and drives it away, then attacks you with a knee to your gut, leaving you gasping.

That's cold to me.

Nevertheless, when I began running seriously, I took it as a point of pride that I would train in any kind of weather. Nothing would stop me. That lasted for years, but those days are now long gone. If I was pressed to say exactly what caused me to change my mind about my all-season running, I would point to my friend Michelle.

Michelle is a very gifted runner and triathlete, and we used to run with a group of other local athletes at 5:30 a.m. every Wednesday at a local track. After a workout one day in the late fall, when the days were getting shorter and the temperatures were dropping, I recalled past years when we ran on the track while the wind blew and the snow fell. I asked Michelle if she was ready to run again in the cold. She said that she wasn't going to do it.

I was struck dumb. "What do you mean?" I finally asked.

"I don't like it, and I'm not going to do it."

I didn't know that was an option. I couldn't believe that an athlete as good as Michelle would just say that she wouldn't do workouts that she didn't like. Stubbornness was one of the shared traits that defined our tribe; we couldn't have led our athletic lives without it. And yet, here she was, saying that she wouldn't do speed-work through the winter *because she didn't want to*. Astonishing.

That's all it took. I stopped running in the cold on dark winter mornings because I didn't want to either. I became an opportunistic runner. I would still run in the winter, but I'd time my workouts for the warmest point of the day. Running is hard, and although I believe in the redemptive value of suffering, I don't believe in needless, unproductive suffering, and that's what being out in the dark cold represents to me.

COLD WEATHER RUNNING

My hatred of the cold isn't just an opinion; it's supported by science. The body handles hot weather by making a bundle of adaptations to keep cool, including increasing blood volume and sweat rate and shunting blood to the surface to shed heat from the core. But in response to the cold, the body does nothing. Nada. When you're cold, all you can do is pile on clothes, drink hot chocolate, and get someplace warm. Or exercise, of course, although even that doesn't seem to do the trick in really frigid weather. Why is this? That seems obvious to me. *Because we're not supposed to be out in the cold.* But that's just my opinion.

I do make an exception for snow, however. I love waking up to discover the world covered in a blanket of white. When I get outdoors, the air is crisp and clean, and the snow crunches under my feet. I head down onto one of the nearby trails, and if I'm lucky, I'll be the first one there, treading on virgin snow. That's when I forgive the winter all of her trespasses.

SNOWMAGEDDON

In February 2010, two back-to-back blizzards combined to dump a record-setting snowfall on the DC area. It was dubbed "Snowmageddon," and it was a once-in-a-lifetime event. I strapped cleats onto my trail-runners, put on a pair of ski goggles, slipped on my ski gloves, and went out to meet my friend Chuck. We found cars were buried in mounds of snow, and people were skiing down snow-covered streets.

Chuck and I made our way slowly down to Rock Creek Park, where our running slowed to a forced hike as we made our way through waist-high snowdrifts. After a few hundred yards, we were exhausted. We made our way back to the road and continued our trek for another hour, at which time we declared victory over the weather and scurried back to our respective homes.

So maybe I don't hate winter. What I dislike is relentless, seemingly endless cold; the kind that wears you down and breaks your spirit. But give me an epic winter day, and I'll be right out there with the hardiest of them.

Whether you love winter running or hate it, you should be mindful about how you approach it.

Dress so that you feel a little chilly at the start of your run. You will always generate a lot of heat when you run—some 75 percent of the energy you metabolize while running goes to warming your body, while only 25 percent goes toward powering muscle contractions. So even on the coldest days, you *will* warm up eventually. If you set out the door wearing enough clothes to feel comfortable, you will overheat once you've warmed up.

Watch your step. Black ice is no joke. I once had my feet sweep out from under me after unknowingly hitting a patch, and like a character in a cartoon, I swung up in the air and then crashed heavily straight down onto my back. I had the breath knocked out of me, and I just lay there for a few moments in the middle of the street, sprawled flat on my back, while my friends wondered if I was down for the count. I got up and kept running, but I learned my lesson: keep your stride shorter when you suspect icy conditions so that you can quickly shift your weight if you lose your footing.

Don't Be Fooled. After you've warmed up, you may come to enjoy your winter run. I hate to say it, after all my complaining about the cold, but I've had some memorable cold weather runs. But think of the cold as being like a wild animal: it may look adorable, but it's still unpredictable and potentially dangerous. As warm as you get, hesitate before taking off any layers, as you can get cold again very quickly. When you are done with your run, don't linger outside; your body temperature drops quickly when you stop moving. Get indoors and get out of your sweaty clothes into something warm and dry.

WARM WEATHER RUNNING

As much as I love running in the summer sun, I know that heat presents challenges and dangers as well.

As I mentioned above, your body has several strategies for dealing with heat, but there's a limit to what it can handle. A good rule of thumb for running in the heat is that when the temperature climbs to about 70 degrees Fahrenheit and above, you should put aside any plans for hard training or racing and just run comfortably. I've never seen temperatures that are too high for running, but I have seen many cases of runners bullying their bodies (that problem again!) into running too hard when they should have been taking it easy.

WHEN HEAT DERAILED A MAJOR MARATHON

It was October 7, 2007. Tens of thousands of runners were lined up for the start of the Chicago Marathon. They were expecting typically cool fall weather, but what they got instead were temperatures in the 70s at the morning start, which soon soared into the upper 80s. Hundreds of runners fell ill, and over 300 had to be picked up by ambulances. One runner died on the course. Hydrants were opened, and air-conditioned buses were provided on the course, but finally the race director called a halt to the race—the first time that a major marathon was suspended after it had begun.

This was a running tragedy in many ways, but I couldn't help thinking that many of the runners who had problems might have pushed themselves too hard on a day when pushing hard should not have been an option. I understand that a race is an opportunity to excel, and that the Chicago Marathon is a bucket-list kind of event for even seasoned runners, but this was one of the times when it would have been crucial for the runners to be smarter than they were brave. "Forget your race goals," I would have told them all. "Go slow. Take walk breaks. Stop off at a convenience store and buy an ice cream. You'll finish eventually, and you'll get to sleep in your own bed tonight."

With that in mind, you should be aware of the warning signs of impending trouble and take the necessary steps to deal with the situation. Heat stroke doesn't just happen; before you collapse, there are a number of stages you pass through as your body begins to strain and shut down. If you pay attention to the signs, you'll be able to take corrective action way before your problem develops into an emergency. Here's what to look for:

- **Dry Skin.** If you are running in the hot sun, you should be sweating. If you are not sweating, you have a problem.
- **Disorientation.** We all can get a little befuddled at some point during a long run, but if you have trouble focusing on basic things, like your address or your mom's phone number (and shame on you if you really don't know it!), you might have a problem.
- **Nausea and Dizziness.** As your body struggles to disperse heat from your core, it will shunt blood away from your stomach and intestines and push it up to the skin surface. The result can be discomfort in your gastro-intestinal tract. Don't ignore it.

If you find yourself experiencing any of these symptoms, a quick response will keep you from getting into real trouble. Here's what you should do:

- **Stop.** Running creates excess heat. If you get too hot, stop running. Simple, right? Slow down to a walk first, and if you don't feel better quickly, stop altogether.
- **Get in the Shade.** On a hot, sunny day, it can be up to 10 degrees cooler in the shade. This may be all the relief that your body needs to get your core temperature under control.
- **Cool Off.** Soak your body down with cold water, paying special attention to the wrists and head. Rub your arms

with ice, if it's available, and put some on the back of your neck.

- **Get Help.** Don't be shy; having a medical emergency is no more embarrassing than having your car conk out. Knock on doors and explain what is going on. Ask for water and ice and, if necessary, for them to call 911.

RUNNING IN THE RAIN

It's a funny thing. I've had some of my best runs when I've gotten caught in a downpour. But if it's raining when I'm ready to step out the door, I won't go. I know that it sounds contradictory, but I'm not the only one who feels this way. I also know that there are many runners who don't mind heading out into the rain, and some who really enjoy it. To each their own, I suppose.

Physiologically, there are factors that support both views. The downsides of running in the rain are that wet socks tend to cause blisters and, since water is an excellent conductor of heat, you can get really cold running in the rain and even risk hypothermia if you are underdressed. Your shoes will also get less traction in the rain, so you risk slipping and falling, especially if you run on brick or across a metal grate.

The upside is that instead of causing you to freeze, rain can cool you off on a warm summer day. Running in the rain can also make an ordinary run feel memorable, even epic. So while a drizzle or soaking rain can be an annoyance, a heavy driving rain can make us feel heroic. Finally, your experience running in the rain will prepare you for possible wet conditions on race day.

Whether you are drawn to or away from running in wet weather, here are some basic tips to follow to make the most of it:

- **It there is thunder—DO NOT RUN.** Runners have been fatally hit by lightning strikes. Do not intentionally put yourself in harm's way. Don't go out in a thunderstorm, and seek shelter if you are caught in one.
- **Dress with water resistant gear, but expect to get wet anyway.** The point of water-resistant gear for a runner isn't really to keep you dry, because you will be soaked by sweat soon enough. It's to keep you warm by keeping the cold rain off of you.
- **A cap could be your most important piece of clothing.** Keeping rain from getting in your eyes will enable you to see where you're going.
- **Pick light shoes with a thin, mesh upper.** If you run in the rain, your shoes will inevitably get wet. The best strategy, then, is not to use heavy, water-resistant shoes that will feel like cement blocks after they get soaked. Instead, use lightweight trainers that will let the water back out after it's gotten in.
- **Splash through puddles.** Do not tiptoe through deep puddles; you'll only get more wet that way. The best technique it to run hard at a deep puddle, with a stomping, fast foot-strike. The force of your step will displace the water, and you will be out of there before it sloshes back. This strategy is best used if you are alone, however, because anyone next to you will get splashed by the spray you've created.

RUNNING WITH PEOPLE

We talked earlier about the tribe of runners and about how, as a runner, you will quickly become a member of this big group. Within this group, though, you will probably have the opportunity to find your own smaller tribe of people to train with. You might meet someone at the office who runs, or you might hit it off with some folks at a local race or organized training run. Maybe these other people share your pace and running goals. Better yet, they seem nice, easy to talk to, and live nearby, so you ask them if they'd like to get together for a run, or they ask you. Either way, you'll find that you are now a member of a pod of runners.

These informal groups are usually focused on training, but if you look closely, you'll see that they also have a significant social component. Even if you only see these people once a week for training runs, they will become a part of your life. You will share stories and come to rely on each other for advice and support, even if it's only during the weekly hour that you hit the roads together.

These training groups are most often informal and ebb and flow naturally as people's situations change. But they will wiggle their way into your life, like a stray puppy with big, soft eyes, and before you know it, they are a permanent fixture. For many people, this personal connection is the best part about running.

There are other people in your training life that you will have to manage as well, however, and these interactions might not be as smooth and effortless as your relationship with your training group.

TRAINING WITH YOUR
SPOUSE OR PARTNER

I have different goals for different workouts. Some workouts are about building endurance, some are about building speed. But some workouts have nothing to do with running; they're about relationships. I use running to strengthen bonds of friendship or to have a little quiet time with my wife.

If you're lucky, these categories will overlap, and your spouse's or partner's training pace and goals coincide with your own. But when that's not the case for me, I temporarily throw my training goals out the window.

The point here is not fitness; it's the bonding. If you are the stronger runner, try to take your partner's feelings into consideration. If you zip ahead, or add miles onto your workout when they've finished, they might feel that what they've done somehow isn't a real workout. Nobody wants to feel like their best isn't good enough, so start and finish with them, and head out on your own either beforehand or afterward to get in your harder work.

It might turn out that your partner doesn't mind if you take off or add more miles; they know themselves, and they don't take any of this personally. In that case, feel free to do what you want. But the point is to be considerate above all else.

BEING A GOOD RUNNING AMBASSADOR

Believe it or not, and like it or not, you are now a role model. Your commitment to running has the power to inspire others to get running shoes and hit the road. These people may be your coworkers, neighbors, and friends, and they may suggest getting together with you to go for a run.

That might sound like a nice idea, but then you think about how far you've come from those first slow, short runs, and the idea of going back and doing that again sounds as appetizing as a dirt sandwich. But there's room in your routine to do a short, slow run, and more importantly, it's a nice thing to do. In all likelihood there were experienced runners who took the time to mentor you when you were just starting out; it's time to pay it back. You don't have to sacrifice all of your runs, or even do this frequently, but as my mother would have said, it won't kill you to help someone out every now and then.

BEING A GOOD CITIZEN

Runners are by nature self-absorbed. Maybe not all of them, but so far, it's true of all the runners I've ever met, and it's certainly true of me.

Having said that, I need to walk it back a little. I don't mean to say that runners are narcissistic (although I'm sure that some of us are). And it doesn't mean that we are uncaring or thought-less (although we can be that way, too). I just mean to say that when we're training, we're focused on what we're doing.

This can occasionally be a problem. As we run, we may startle people, run red lights, and even accidentally brush against pedestrians, or worse still, bang into someone. Usually, we don't stop; we just wave our hand in apology or shout "I'm sorry" over our shoulder as we zip past. Because, hey, we're working on our pace.

I've made a big effort to stop being *that guy*, and you should, too. First of all, it's rude, and as I've tried to teach my son, what-ever your disagreement is with anyone, there's never an excuse for being rude. These are people, not just roadblocks or speed bumps.

Second, whether we like it or not, each of us represents our sport when we're out there, and every time we make someone angry, we've just created an enemy for runner-friendly infrastructure. Want a bike and run lane on your street? Then act like a responsible member of your community, and the chances are better that your voice will be heard.

So this is how I run these days: Think of how you would like someone to treat your grandmother on the street, and then treat everyone the same way. I call out to walkers when I'm coming up behind them and slow down so I don't startle them. I obey traffic lights (although you might still see me zip across a street through a red light in the early morning if there is absolutely no one anywhere around). I smile and say thanks if someone moves out of my way, and I wave to everyone who says something nice and encouraging.

I've been surprised at how it's paid off. People respond to kindness with kindness. In return for my thoughtfulness, I've gotten waves and good wishes, and because I often run the same route at the same time of day, I've established something with the people I see regularly. Maybe not exactly a friendship, but at least a friendly familiarity.

All of this has made my runs more pleasant, which is enough of a good reason to keep being friendly. But I also like to think that I've done some small service to the entire running community by adding to the number of people who are favorably inclined to our tribe.

THINKING ABOUT YOUR ROUTE

I like trivia, and I like history. On my runs, these two interests often come together. I like to find out interesting things about the buildings and places that I pass on my run, and if you're running with me, chances are that I will share them with you.

Recently, during a workout with a local running class I teach, I rolled out yet another strange factoid about a monument that we were passing. One student asked why I like these little bits of information.

It was a fair question. I said that I look on each little fact as being like a piece in a jigsaw puzzle. The more I can learn, the more pieces of the puzzle that I find a place for, the more I can see what the entire picture might look like, and I come just a tiny bit closer to understanding the world around me.

But some days I want none of this; I just want to run in the woods or on a path along the river. In my imagination, I am no longer in a 21st-century city; I am a hunter tracking game with a spear or a bow and arrow. If I am fast enough and do not stop, I might yet eat tonight. If I falter, if I fail to catch my quarry, I will put my whole tribe at risk. So I run faster.

Or sometimes I just want to see something new, whether it's a trail in a park or an unexplored neighborhood or street. Just something different.

Adventure and curiosity. To me, that's the heart of running.

Like all long-term relationships, my connection to running can sometimes feel stale. Instead of feeling the thrill I experienced when I first discovered long-distance running, I sometimes feel boredom and impatience. Love becomes duty, and my passion becomes a chore.

If you're like me, I encourage you to seek out new routes. Explore on foot, or find suggestions online, but be willing to feed your sense of play. Running, after all, should be about having fun.

Of course, you may completely disagree with me on this. You may be the kind of runner who has a favorite route and sticks with it, weekend after weekend, month after month, year after year. Some of my favorite running and cycling buddies fall into this category. And I get it: they enjoy comparing their workouts and like to be able to run without worrying about getting lost. As they come to know every pothole or rock, their runs becoming like visits with an old friend.

The bottom line of this chapter is that your task is to think about where you most like to run, whom—if anyone—you like to run with, and when you like to run. By asking yourself these questions, you will become aware of your preferences and be able to make purposeful choices.

RUNNING ON SAND

The extra effort needed to run on sand can make for a more intense, effective workout, with the added bonus that the softness of the sand should make the old knees happy. Right?

Well, sort of. It's true that sand is a lower-impact running surface than concrete, asphalt, or even trails. But that softness also creates a problem: shifting sand changes the mechanics of the push-off phase of your running stride, so instead of landing on your heel and forefoot and pushing off as you normally would, your foot sinks into the sand and moves around more than it would on solid ground, causing more flexing of the ankle and arch.

While this movement isn't necessarily bad—and in fact can lead to added strength—it is something new for your body to deal with. Until it adjusts and adapts, the risk of injury is elevated. Run a little too far, and you may suddenly find yourself with a sore Achilles tendon.

Another potential problem is the fact that sand can act as an abrasive. Running barefoot on sand can lead to blisters and raw spots if your feet aren't given time to toughen up with calluses.

Feel discouraged? Don't be. With a little planning, you can head out for that beach run. Keep these tips in mind:

- **Scale back and add miles incrementally.** You might be used to a 10-mile training run on the roads, but don't plan to suddenly do that at the beach. Start with just a few miles and add more distance slowly—no more than a mile from each workout to the next.

- **Start on the road.** If you need or want a longer run than would be feasible on the sand, start out on a road and end your workout with a few sand miles.

- **Wear shoes and run close to the water.** Wet sand provides a slightly more compact surface than dry sand. Wearing shoes will protect the skin of your feet from getting rubbed raw.

- **Gauge your run by effort level, not pace.**
  Running on sand is harder than running on
  roads. Just as you would not expect to run
  uphill at the same pace you run on the flats,
  don't expect to keep your usual training
  pace during your sand run.

CHAPTER THREE

CROSS-TRAINING

Cross-training can be a difficult subject to bring up because I know that there are many runners who disagree with me about this or who don't want to talk about it.

I get it. Runners want to run. None of us get into running so that we can spend more time in the gym. We love being out on the roads and trails. Even running indoors on the tread-mill—derisively called the *dread*mill—is often looked upon with disdain, so you can imagine what runners generally think of every other piece of fitness equipment. In some wonderful and miraculous way, running makes our days better in ways we can't even fully explain. None of that happens for us in a gym or on a stationary bike—at least not in the same way, even on the best of days.

I feel the same way, but nonetheless I'm going to try to convince you to spend some of your exercise time away from running and focus on a nonrunning workout. Don't frown and skip this chapter; I'm not trying to force anyone to do anything they don't want to do. I just ask you to keep an open mind and think about the things we're about to discuss.

START WITH THE BIG PICTURE

The best way to approach your fitness for any sport is to make yourself as broadly strong and healthy as possible, and then add sport-specific training.

Look at it this way: your fitness is like a college education. You should take your generally required classes before you declare a major, presumably because this will make you a more well-rounded, critically thinking person who is then better positioned to excel in your particular area of interest.

The benefit of taking this approach to your fitness is twofold. First, by building a body that is strong overall, you will reduce the risk of injury from running because you will not have any weak links in your movement chain. Weakness in one or more muscle groups is responsible for many typical running injuries.

To get better at anything, including running, you need to do that thing. That's called *specificity of movement*. If you want to get better at table tennis, you need to practice table tennis. All the swimming in the world won't help you. It will make you healthier, but it won't make you better at table tennis. Writers have to write, singers need to sing, and runners need to run.

But if all you do is run, you open yourself up to injury because you've left important muscles undertrained. Running is wonderful for improving your cardiovascular fitness, and it builds strong calves, hamstrings, and gluteus maximus muscles, but it doesn't do as much for the core muscles or the quadriceps.

Whenever you leave a muscle group undertrained, the load falls on other muscle groups to pick up the slack. These other muscles overcompensate, which puts them at risk of strain and injury. Essentially, you have planted a landmine, and one day, maybe not this year or the next, but eventually, the odds are that it will blow up on you.[7]

Here's an example. Running is mostly a back-of-body movement. The gluteus maximus and hamstring muscles are the driving force behind running, and they grow strong from running. The quadriceps muscles at the front of your legs are used in running mostly to absorb the impact of foot-strike. Running doesn't strengthen these muscles quite as much.

The result, for many runners, is that they have underpowered quads. The problem is that quad muscles are also largely responsible for holding the kneecaps in proper alignment. If the quads aren't doing their job because they lack the strength to do so, the kneecaps will slide around, resulting in pain and inflammation on the front of the knee. When you see your doctor or orthopedist because you can no longer run without pain, they will tell you that you have patellar tendinitis or patellofemoral pain syndrome, commonly known as runner's knee, and they will tell you to start doing exercises that strengthen your quads.

---

7 See, for example, Ajit M. W. Chaudhari et al., "Reducing Core Stability Influences Lower Extremity Biomechanics in Novice Runners," *Medicine & Science in Sports Exercise* 52, no. 6 (June 2020): 1347–53. This is not to diminish the role of many other risk factors in causing running injuries, such as overuse, but lack of core strength is a very big factor.

This injury, and so many others, could be avoided by maintaining the kind of balanced fitness that results from cross-training.

Further, if all you do is run, you leave yourself open to repetitive stress injuries. Economists call this the law of diminishing returns. Things we enjoy doing may provide us with happiness and improve us in some way—up to a point. After that, the benefits begin to level off and negative consequences set in. Your favorite food goes from being delicious in the first serving, to distasteful in the fourth serving, to causing stomach upset and nausea in the eighth serving.

So it is with running. The ideal number of miles to run per week varies with every runner and is dependent on the runner's goals, training, and injury history, as well as their inherited physiology and biomechanics. But every runner has a sweet spot where their weekly running supports good health and performance while keeping them injury free. For many people, that number is somewhere around 30 to 40 miles per week. But if they step over that invisible marker, things begin breaking down. Cross-training would allow them to continue training and improving fitness without entering that negative zone.

The second benefit of cross-training is a bit more esoteric. It has less to do with your running and instead focuses on your overall approach to life.

I believe that life should be an adventure and that fitness is not a goal in itself, but simply a tool that enables you to seek out those adventures, allowing you to live your life to the fullest. Having fitness without any adventures seems to me like having a sports car that you never take out of the garage. Sure, it might look nice, and just having it might give you some pleasure, but really, what's the point? Take it out on the road and see what it can do!

You have a great interest and love for running. That's why you're reading this book. But you are many things in addition to being a runner, and perhaps there are other adventures you would also like to try. How about circumnavigating Manhattan Island by kayak? Or climbing up the cable trail on Half Dome in Yosemite National Park? Or just taking a yoga class or joining your friends for a round of golf? All of these activities should be within reach with some specific training because you have already developed good overall fitness.

It might sound like something you would see in a fortune cookie, but that doesn't make it less true: to live your best life, prepare your body to do anything you may ever want to do. Then, when you get that crazy idea, just fine-tune your training for that specific challenge.

If it's true that history predicts destiny, then this is also the approach that our bodies have evolved to take. Exercise theorists and evolutionary biologists have posited that our species evolved to be able to run great distances, which enabled them to eventually outrun game that could not match our endurance. This gave our ancestors a readily available source of protein, which enabled them to grow bigger brains, which, millions of years later, has resulted in my teenage son Alex spending too much time on his smartphone. In fact, running itself might have triggered adaptations in our brain that improved our chances of survival.[8]

---

8 Jay Schulkin, "Evolutionary Basis of Human Running and Its Impact on Neural Function," *Frontiers in Systems Neuroscience*, July 11, 2016. doi: 10.3389/fnsys.2016.00059.

But there's more to the story than just that. Running was not the only activity that enabled our ancestors to survive and thrive. As upright animals with freely swinging arms, at the end of which were hands with opposable thumbs, our ancestors were able to climb and lift and twist and reach. They invented farming, put animals to work, and built homes and villages. They did all of these things and more because their bodies enabled them to do so, and by doing these things they improved the health and fitness of their bodies.

Put simply, we were all born to move in many ways. When we live in accordance with the way our bodies have evolved to move, we create the environment for healthier living.

If you were already a fitness generalist and then got into running, you're ahead of the game. I've known runners like this, and they defy expectations because their fitness baseline is already so high. One runner I know completed a marathon on a base of training that I would have called insufficient—except that he was already exceptionally fit before he even began his marathon training.

If you're not a fitness generalist and are new to running, this is a good time to add cross-training to your program. By doing that now, you will avoid many of the problems that long-time runners often experienced before they added cross-training to their routine.

If you're a long-time runner, this is still a good time to start cross-training. Many of us developed our cross-training program as a direct result of recovering from various injuries over the years. When the injuries subsided, the cross-training routines that helped heal us remained, and we stuck with them to reduce the risk of reinjuring ourselves.

So there's really no bad time to begin cross-training. You will start reaping the benefits whenever you begin. To borrow a popular phrase, just do it.

WHAT IS CROSS-TRAINING?

Now that I have, hopefully, gotten you to at least consider cross-training, let's take a closer look at what that means. We'll begin by defining what cross-training actually is.

Cross-training for runners is simply any exercise that is not running. This covers a lot of ground, so let's break it down further. Cross-training can be divided into aerobic, or cardiovascular, cross-training, and anaerobic, or strength, cross-training.

AEROBIC CROSS-TRAINING

Aerobic cross-training involves any repetitive rhythmic activity that raises your heart rate for an extended period of time. This includes cycling, rowing, swimming, fast walking, hiking, and a wide range of other activities. All of them will trigger many of the same kinds of physiological changes that running does:

- Improving your heart health by lowering your blood pressure and resting heart rate while improving your heart's ability to pump more blood more efficiently.
- Raising your intake and distribution of oxygen and enhancing your body's ability to deliver oxygen to working muscles, called your VO_2 max
- Reducing your risk of developing diabetes and certain cancers.

Aerobic cross-training will also reduce the amount of pounding that you impose on your body, because most of these modes of training are either non- or very low-impact.

Also, many of them, especially cycling, will strengthen muscle groups that do not improve from running, but which will benefit your running, such as those quadriceps muscles we just talked about.

Aerobic cross-training not only helps runners to avoid injury, but it also helps build even greater fitness. It enables runners to build their endurance without adding more miles onto their tired legs. So instead of taking a rest day or doing a shorter recovery run on weekends between long runs, you can do a long cross-training session. After all, your heart doesn't care what you do to keep it fit; all aerobic exercise counts.

To me, this is like stealing fitness. You can rest your sore and aching muscles and joints but still work on improving your aerobic conditioning. Then you'll come back strong and eager for your next running workout.

This is not a training guide, so we won't talk about how to specifically incorporate aerobic cross-training into your routine. That would be a book unto itself.[9] But to think like a runner, you should consider adding some aerobic cross-training to your weekly workout routine.

ANAEROBIC CROSS-TRAINING

Anaerobic cross-training, or strength training, includes exercises that use short, repeated sets of movements to build strength in

---

9 Which, actually, I did write: *Smart Marathon Training* (Velo Press).

the skeletal muscles.[10] This involves moving your body against resistance, which may take the form of free weights like dumb-bells or barbells; exercise machines, which rely on stacks of plates or pistons to generate resistance; elastic bands or cables; or even your own bodyweight, as when you do push-ups or pull-ups.

This is not the place to set out a complete strength-training program; that would also be another subject for a book unto itself.[11] What I want to do here instead is present a way of thinking about strength training that will help you specifically as a runner.

TO GYM OR NOT TO GYM?

Once a runner agrees to cross-train, their next question usually is whether they need to join a gym.

The quick answer is no.

Not that there's anything wrong with joining a fitness center. When you belong to a gym, you'll have access to much more equipment than you could likely ever afford to own or manage to fit into your living space. You'll also probably have easy access to a wide range of health professionals,

---

10 Interestingly, strength training has also been shown to also have a beneficial effect on heart health by lowering blood pressure. See Rafael Ribeiro Correia et al., "Strength Training for Arterial Hypertension Treatment: A Systematic Review and Meta-Analysis of Randomized Clinical Trials," *Scientific Reports* 13, article 201, January 5, 2023. https://doi.org/10.1038/s41598-022-26583-3"10.1038/s41598-022-26583-3.

11 Which I have also written: *Quick Strength for Runners* (Velo Press).

such as personal trainers, massage therapists, and certified nutritionists.

But you can fit a strength training routine easily into your own living space with a limited amount of equipment. If you do a core workout, yoga, or other type of bodyweight workout, all you need is a workout mat.

To expand your home workout options, all you need to do is add a few pieces of inexpensive equipment. These would be a good start:

- **Stability Ball.** This adds an element of instability when you do exercises sitting on it, lying back on it, or when you prop your feet up on it while lying on the floor. Instability engages the core, so you'll be improving your balance and your core strength as you work out. We'll talk about this again shortly.

- **Resistance Bands.** These allow you to add resistance to your movements in a wide variety of exercises and are light enough to go with you on vacation or anywhere else you go.

- **Ab Wheel.** This might be the best return on investment in the world of fitness. Done properly, this simple tool gives your abdominals a great workout.

- **BOSU.** Like the stability ball, this piece of equipment provides an unstable platform for exercise that will help you engage your core effectively. Any exercise that you can do sitting, lying down, or standing, you can do from atop the BOSU.

- **Wobble Board.** This is another tool to use to destabilize yourself while working out. We'll talk about this again shortly.
- **Stacking Dumbbells.** This is a higher-priced piece of equipment, but in terms of ease of use, flexibility, and small footprint, it pays for itself. Basic sets offer a range of 6 to 24 pounds, and advanced sets double that capacity.

Exercise in general can be described as the introduction of certain kinds of stimuli that are intended to trigger an adaptation response in the body. In other words, if you push your body out of its comfort zone in a calculated way, it will respond by resculpting itself to meet the challenge. This is why we exercise, and this is how we get better.

The way the body responds—and changes—depends on the nature of the stimulus. In general, if you work out with greater resistance and low repetitions you will build more muscle strength and size, while if you use lighter weights and more repetitions you will develop more muscle endurance.[12]

---

12 Your response to strength training will depend not only on the way in which you train, but also on your genetic make-up. There's a coaching phrase that applies here: anatomy is destiny. That means your ultimate success in training for any sport will depend largely on your body type. But remember: even though your genetics might place limits on what you can achieve, everyone improves with training and practice.

As runners, we're less concerned with strength and muscle size than we are with functionality. While we might all like to look good on the beach, our muscles are not for show; as runners we expect them to work for us when we're running. With that in mind, we can set specific guidelines for our training.

First, we will aim to engage the core as much as possible. The core—all the muscles from the upper legs to the ribcage, front, sides, and back—is the foundation of the body. All movement rests in having a strong core to maintain stability as the limbs move out into space and as your center of gravity shifts.

Second, we will aim for multi-joint movements as much as possible. This will ensure that instead of simply trying to get a specific muscle stronger and bigger, you will engage them in more complex movements that might mimic what you do in real life. This is the essence of functionality. We'll talk more about this in a moment.

Third, we won't try to push big resistance. Many runners fear that strength training will involve lifting very heavy weights, but that's not necessarily true. There's nothing wrong with having a goal of bench-pressing twice your body weight; it's just that doing so will not help your running. Tap into your endurance and aim to build lean muscle mass by choosing to lift lighter weights and doing more repetitions.

OUR GUIDING PRINCIPLE

With all this in mind, we can now set out our guiding principle for strength training:

Our goal in strength training is to build our library of kinesthetic sense by engaging our brain in problem solving.

There's a lot going on in that sentence. Read it again.

This is the prime directive that you should keep in mind every time you start your workout. Write it on a slip of paper and put it in your wallet; write it on your bathroom mirror; put it on a note on your refrigerator door. It's a big one.

Now let's break it down.

Kinesiology is the science of body movement. This is what exercise physiologists study when they ponder human biomechanics. Kinesthetic sense, then, is our own awareness and control over our body movements. This is linked to proprioception, which is the body's awareness of itself in space, especially in relation to force and motion, and to interoception, which is your awareness of your own body parts. When combined, these sensory perceptions enable you to feel your muscles contracting, and know where you are moving.

THE BIOLOGY OF EXERCISE

We're going to take a break for a moment here and briefly go back to biology class. Don't panic; our visit won't be long.

We are all born with an incredibly dense neural network. The brain itself is composed of about ten billion neurons, each of which is connected to ten thousand other neurons. These neurons are information messengers; they transmit information to the brain and relay orders from the brain to the body. Some of these instructions happen autonomously, as when your body regulates your heart rate or your temperature. But some instructions are voluntary, such as when you decide to lift your arm.

A neural pathway is the connection formed from one neuron to another to enable movement of information, called a neurotransmission. Neuroplasticity describes the way in which the brain creates neural pathways in response to experience. It was long thought that this process takes place only during our early development, when we all learned to walk and talk. But it's now understood that neuroplasticity takes place throughout adulthood as well.[13] In other words, we can all still learn how to move our bodies in new ways.

Research has also shown that exercise and physical activity can stimulate neuroplasticity in adults, leading to a wide range of benefits, including improved memory, cognitive function, and cardiovascular adjustments.[14] That means that when we exercise, we are essentially rewiring our neural network to improve our health and fitness.

Stay with me; we're almost at the finish line.

Repetitive motion can induce neural plasticity and strengthen the resulting neural network. In other words, the more you practice a movement, the better you are able to do it. That's why you keep doing your piano drills and practicing your tennis serve. As the saying goes, practice makes perfect.

But it doesn't end there. When you create that new neural pathway, it sticks. You can stop moving your body in that way, but you will have a quicker re-adaptation if you get back to

---

13 Alvaro Pascual-Leone et al., "The Plastic Human Brain Cortex," *Annual Review of Neuroscience* 28 (July 2005): 377–401.

14 Lisete C. Michelini and Javier E. Stern, "Exercise-Induced Neuronal Plasticity in Central Autonomic Networks: Role in Cardiovascular Control," *Experimental Physiology* 94, no. 9 (September 2009): 947–60.

using that skill. This is called "savings," and it is why you can ride a bicycle after not having done it in years.[15]

Now back to analyzing our guiding principle.

That neural network that we just described is our library of kinesthetic sense. When we try a new movement, our brain learns how to do it, and it keeps the ability to do that movement. With our billions of neurons linked to all our skeletal muscles, we are born with the capacity to engage our bodies in an incredibly wide range of movements. We only need to try.

I think of it like this: our neural network is like a road map of a big city. In the particular city in which each of us lives, there are thousands of alleys, roads, streets, and highways. Most of us will travel only a small portion of them in our lifetime, but the routes we regularly take become ingrained in our minds. Sometimes we may leave our place of work or a supermarket and then find ourselves at the front door of our home, with little memory of how we got there. We just moved on autopilot, letting our conscious mind deal with other things while we made our way home.

Imagine now that your goal is to visit as many alleys, roads, and streets in your city as possible. You will see new neighborhoods and discover new shops, meet new people, and, most important, learn new ways to get around. You will discover useful shortcuts, and if there's a traffic jam, you will know how to avoid it.

---

15 Sofia M. Landi et al., "One Week of Motor Adaptation Induces Structural Changes in the Primary Motor Cortex That Predict Long-Term Memory One Year Later," *Journal of Neuroscience* 31, no. 33 (August 17, 2011): 11808–13.

This is the goal we have for our bodies. We want to create these new neural pathways—these new routes through the city that is our neural network—in order to be able to move more effectively, efficiently, and safely.

This is the essence of functional training: to exercise in a way that not just makes us look better, but also helps us move better throughout the day. To build our library of kinesthetic sense.

With that as our goal, the question is, How do we get there? That involves the other part of our guiding principle: engaging our brains in problem solving.

Every time we move in a new way, our brain has to figure out how to engage our muscles to move our body the way we want it to and to maintain balance while doing so. That's not an easy task, but it's one that our brain is used to doing, and that it has done thousands of times before. From the moment that you learned how to roll over in the crib, to when you first walked, to when you learned to drive a car, your brain has repeatedly learned how to move your body in new, complex ways.

That process doesn't have to stop. If we ask it now to move in a way that's unfamiliar, it will, sooner or later, figure it out, and then add that movement to its library of movements. Our goal, then, is to continue to challenge our brain in that way; to do new things in new ways so that our brain will adapt and learn.

This approach to exercise is not only more useful than doing the same old thing over and over again; it's also more fun. Exercise is by its nature repetitive, but that doesn't mean it always has to be boring. If you're bored, then your body is bored, and nothing new is happening. While all safe, appropriate movement is beneficial, let's aim to do the ones that will give us the biggest bang for our buck: the more challenging ones.

PUTTING IT INTO ACTION

You might be thinking right now that, sure, this all makes sense, but how hard is it going to be to figure out how to apply this principle? The answer is not very hard at all. There are two strategies that we can use to help us out.

Reduce Stability

The first is to aim to reduce stability whenever you can while working out. When you're feeling wobbly, your brain has to work to figure out how to keep from toppling over. It does that by engaging the muscles in your core that will help you to regain control and remain upright. In doing so, your brain will strengthen your core muscles, which will help you with your running, and establish a new neural pathway.

We can reduce stability in several easy ways. One is to remove a support, and another is to remove the visual cues that help you maintain balance.

Try this: stand up. Now, pick one foot off the floor. You have now removed one of the supports that your body relies on to stay upright. Perhaps you are wobbling a bit. That's natural. After some time, your brain will figure out how to make this work, and you will wobble less.

Now, try closing your eyes while you hold one foot off the ground. You'll find that this is much harder. You may find that even standing on both feet with your eyes closed is disorienting. That's because your brain relies on visual cues, along with core strength and your inner ear, to maintain balance. Without your visual cues to rely on, your brain will be forced to strengthen its neural pathways to the muscles it will use to keep you balanced.

Try to apply this strategy during your strength workout. Any exercise that you would do standing up, try doing it while standing on one leg, or with your eyes closed, or both. It's surprisingly difficult. Stick with it; you'll get better.

Another strategy is to lift weights unilaterally, or asymmetrically. This means that instead of doing an exercise with a dumbbell in each hand, you work one arm at a time using a single dumbbell. The result is that you will be unbalanced, as your body will have to fight being pulled to the side where you are holding the weight.

There are also several pieces of inexpensive exercise equipment that can help you reduce stability. We briefly mentioned them earlier: the wobble board and the stability ball.

The name "wobble board" gives away its purpose. It's a large flat disk that has a half dome underneath. When you stand on the flat side, you will be perched on the dome, which you will quickly discover is a very precarious place to be. As you struggle to stay atop the board, you will be building strength and balance. Now try to do exercises while standing on the wobble board. Squats, shoulder presses, really any exercise is much harder to do when you're not standing on solid ground.

The inflatable stability ball is another tool that you should consider. As we mentioned earlier, any exercise that you perform lying back or sitting down on a bench or on the floor can be performed from atop the stability ball, and its roundness will force you to work harder.

Make It Complicated

The second strategy that we rely on to hit our goal is to make each exercise as complicated as possible. Simple exercises are those that require the movement of only a single joint. Bicep curls, for example, just require you to bend your elbow. Complex exercises, however, require the movement of two or more joints. A dumbbell row, for example, requires you to use your elbow and shoulder joints to pull the weight up toward your ribs. That uses two joints. A squat engages our hip, knee, and ankle joints, and a squat with a shoulder press . . . well, you get the idea.

When you make exercises more complicated, you work more muscles, which will make your workout more time efficient. For example, if you do a bicep curl, as we mentioned above, you will be primarily working the muscles in the front of your arm. But if you do a row, you'll be working those muscles as well as the muscles of your upper back and rear shoulder. You will be getting more done in the same amount of time.

You will also be moving more functionally. In the real world, we rarely use only one joint when we move. We use many joints when we bend and twist and jump and, yes, run. By adding additional functionality to our workouts in this way, we are encouraging our brain to create new neural pathways that could help support all of our complex movements, including running.

This is where you can bring your own creativity into play. You can find many challenging exercises in books and online, but by applying these strategies, you may be able to create new exercises of your own. When you challenge yourself in this way, you will be improving your fitness for running and whatever else you might try doing, but you could also be doing something else: having fun. I've had clients laugh when they wobbled and tipped over, and then flash a big smile when they succeed at whatever new challenge we've taken up.

This isn't to be taken lightly; fun matters. If you're having fun, your body is having fun. There's an old saying among trainers and coaches that applies here: the best exercises and workouts are the ones you like to do. Go find them.

A final word about these strategies and our overall goal: never try a new movement that might be unsafe or can unreasonably raise the risk of injury. I say unreasonably because all movement can lead to injury, but there are some that would be, in my opinion, foolish to try. We should only try new exercises that require us to engage our muscles in a way that improves health and fitness. A client of mine once put this well. "Any new movement can be difficult," he said, "but we should only do the ones that can also be productive." Exactly so.

CHAPTER FOUR

RUNNING FORM

Mind is everything. Muscle—pieces of rubber. All that I am, I am because of my mind.

—Paavo Nurmi,
nine-time Olympic gold medalist

It's a sad truth: no one teaches us how to run when we're young. It's assumed that we already know how to do it, since we all started unsteadily running around when we were two years old or so. Instead, they give us piano, swimming, or tennis lessons. But although most people run, few do it correctly. There is a right way to run, and that should be taught to us when we are young.

But it's never too late to learn. By engaging our minds to understand the mechanics of running, we will be able to control our movements and run purposefully. We will become true *athletes*.

THE BIOMECHANICS OF RUNNING

Let's begin by looking at how running works. The movement involves the swinging of your arms and legs, mostly all on a single plane. Your arms swing back and forth, and your legs pump up and forward and down and back. There's no stepping to the outside or swinging laterally. A runner should be able to easily run down a long narrow corridor without ever touching the walls.

Now, let's take a closer look at your leg motion. It would be helpful if you think of your leg going around in a circle, as your foot does when you ride a bicycle. Each part of this circle is a distinct phase of the running motion:

- Knee lift
- Leg extension
- Foot-strike
- Push-off

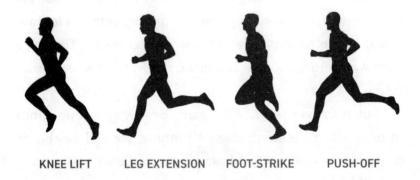

KNEE LIFT   LEG EXTENSION   FOOT-STRIKE   PUSH-OFF

The first phase, lift-off, is familiar to us. It's the starting movement of running, when you drive your leg up and your opposite arm forward. This is an explosive movement, creating momentum that lifts your body up off the ground and propels it forward.

Leg extension is when your body prepares your leg for landing. Your lower leg will automatically swing out, like a door on a hinge, and you will automatically lift your toes up—an action called dorsiflexion—as you prepare for contact with the ground.

Foot-strike occurs when you land. Your body has two chores to do at this point: absorb the shock of impact and prepare for push-off. Your quadriceps, the muscles on the front of your thighs, take much of the brunt of landing. If you jump up and down in front of a full-length mirror, you'll see how your quads shake on landing as they do their job.

Your foot takes a lot of this force as well, as the arch flattens and the foot rolls to disperse the impact force, an action call pronation. Then the second chore of the foot kicks in: it has to stiffen into a lever for push-off.

This is where the magic happens. It's actually the most important phase of running, because this is where you propel your body forward and *run*. The other phases are just preparation and recovery for this moment. Your glutes engage, pushing your hips forward as your foot pushes back. Finally, your hamstrings engage in the follow-through to your push-off, and you kick up your heel and prepare to repeat the cycle.

Running, then, isn't a smooth glide forward; it's a series of rapid accelerations as you push off, and brief decelerations as you glide through the air.

Looked at another way, running is a complex series of movements, requiring activation of many different muscles in a specific sequence. When each muscle group involved is doing its job properly and your movement is done correctly, you will run smoothly and efficiently.

If some muscles are not doing their job because they are underpowered or you are not moving your body properly, then your form becomes compromised. As a result, muscles and tendons get overstressed, and injuries can occur.

We know this intuitively. We've all seen the people who make running look easy. We don't know exactly what's going on, but we know it looks beautiful. They look like true athletes.

And then there are other runners who look like they're doing something very wrong. We can't quite put our fingers on it, but their running looks stilted, even painful.

If we were all versed in the biomechanics of running, we would be able to explain precisely why someone does or does not look good while running. This is exactly what physical therapists do when they do a gait analysis. They have a checklist of problems that they look for, and recommendations to make if they see those problems occurring. While I do recommend having your gait analyzed by a trained professional, we can still make some improvements in our running form right now.

HOW TO IMPROVE YOUR RUNNING FORM

The first thing we need to do is to create self-awareness about our running. We talked earlier about associative and dissociative running. As you recall, the difference is between focusing on what your body is doing as an associative runner, versus trying to distract yourself during running as a dissociative runner. To become better runners—to learn how to run correctly—we're going to have to spend some time being associative.

Before we review the biomechanics of running, however, let's talk about some of the limits of this discussion. I'm reminded now of the Serenity Prayer. Perhaps you're familiar with it; I've seen it painted on plaques and embroidered on throw pillows all across our country. It was written by the American theologian Reinhold Niebuhr, and it goes like this:

> God, grant me the serenity to accept the things I cannot change,
> the courage to change the things I can,
> and the wisdom to know the difference.[16]

This prayer has particular relevance to runners. There are things about our bodies that we cannot change. We are the beneficiaries and victims of our genetics and of our life experiences. These attributes will affect our running, and all we can do is accommodate them and work with them as best we can. If you have flat feet or high arches, for example, you'll need to buy the appropriate running shoes to compensate for those characteristics. I can't simply tell you not to be that way.

There are many other aspects of our running, however, that are within our control. These are the things that, as associative runners, we focus on. With practice and patience, we can make improvements in these areas and become faster, more efficient, and more injury-resistant runners.

This doesn't mean that you can't listen to your music or your favorite podcast while you run. There will still be room

---

16 "Prayer for Serenity," https://www.marquette.edu/faith/prayer-serenity.php#:~:text=God%2C%20grant%20me%20the%20serenity,wisdom%20to%20know%20the%20difference.

for being dissociative. Paying attention to your running form should not be a very time-consuming or exhausting chore, at least not after you get used to it.

Think of being an associative runner as if you're driving a car. You should pay attention to a number of things as you drive, both inside and outside of your vehicle. Most of the time you'll look straight ahead, checking for stop signs and traffic lights, and monitoring pedestrians and other cars. But you'll do more than that; you'll also glance at your speedometer and maybe your fuel gauge, and you'll look at the rearview and both side-view mirrors. You'll glance back over your shoulder as you change lanes. You'll do all of this repeatedly as you drive, perhaps every minute or so, depending on the road conditions.

You won't, however, be very anxious and tense about this. At least, I hope not. You won't hold the steering wheel in a death grip and grit your teeth. Unless you've spotted a problem like an erratic driver up ahead or a traffic jam, you'll be relaxed as you drive. You can listen to the radio or even let your mind wander a little, but you won't stop looking around and paying attention.

So, too, with your running. We'll aim for that level of relaxed self-awareness.

RUNNING TIPS

Now we're ready to talk about what you should be focusing on as you run. Think of each of these points as being items on a checklist. Just as you have that checklist for driving, we're going to develop a checklist of items that you should review every few minutes as you run.

RUN QUIETLY

This is the most important advice that anyone can ever give you on running form: try to keep your foot-strike as quiet as possible. Run silently.

Here's why: the second biggest predictor of injury is impact force. (The first one is a previous injury. You may heal, but unfortunately, the body never forgets.) The more force you generate when you land, the more pressure you put on your body, and the higher the risk that something will break down.

How do you run quietly? Experiment and see what works. It really won't be too difficult. The important thing, though, is to get in the habit of *listening* to your footsteps so you can make those adjustments as needed.

ENGAGE YOUR CORE

The deepest layer of muscle in your midsection, beneath the beach-ready six-pack and the love handles, is the transverse abdominal (TVA). This is a lateral sheath of muscle that wraps around your midsection. Its job is to support and stabilize your body as you move.

Think of your TVA as being like a piece of construction equipment. If you've ever looked closely at the machines at a construction site, you might have noticed that they often have big metal arms that stick out from their sides and are planted on the ground. These arms help keep the base stable so that other moving parts—like the crane arm or the shovel—can move without tipping the whole contraption over.

Your TVA serves the same purpose as those metal arms. It keeps your body balanced as your arms and legs move. Running, after all, is an inherently unbalanced activity. You never have both feet on the ground, which means your body is always on the verge of tipping over. A strong core, and a strong TVA in particular, will prevent this. Your body will engage your TVA automatically as you move, but we're aiming to help your body out by engaging it consciously.

So how do you engage your TVA? It's easy. Stand in a relaxed position, with one hand resting lightly on your stomach. Now keep your hand steady as you suck in your stomach, away from your hand. Don't pull in too much; just enough to break contact between your hand and your belly. You should feel a gentle clenching of your stomach muscles. That's your TVA being contracted.

You should aim to activate your TVA whenever you run, and even as you move through life, especially when you squat down and when you bend over. Your TVA is tasked with helping support your back and keeping you in balance whenever you move, so by engaging it consciously, you're helping it do its job.

To strengthen the TVA, you need to not just work your abdominal muscles, but to also do balance exercises. Yoga in particular can help with this. I used to be fearful of looking foolish in class, which I know now that I shouldn't have cared about. But as I worked to improve my balance and abdominal strength in the gym and at home, I found that I had laid the groundwork for being a yogi. I now do at least some yoga almost every day, and I even enjoy it.

TAKE SHORT, QUICK STEPS

Speed comes not from long strides, but from short, quick steps. That's because, as we just discussed, propulsion only comes from push-off, and time spent in the air during a long stride is time spent decelerating. Therefore, the more times you can push off per minute, the greater propulsion you'll generate. It's like stepping on the gas pedal more frequently while driving.

Exercise physiologists have found that the ideal running cadence, or the number of total steps taken per minute, is around 180 steps per minute. That's 3 steps per second. At that rate, you'll have your weight fully on your planted foot when it's directly below you, which means you'll not just be pushing off more frequently, but you'll also avoid overstriding and heel-striking. That's because your quick stride will not give you enough time to throw your foot far out in front of you.

This is important for avoiding injury because your heels are very bad at absorbing impact forces on foot-strike. Instead, they transmit those forces up the chain to your knees, hips, and back. If that doesn't hurt immediately, it probably will soon, and then comes injury and a layoff from running.

As the infomercials say, But wait! There's more.

When you overstride—when your foot is planted in front of you rather than directly below you on full landing—you are also running less efficiently. That's because of Newtonian physics: every application of force creates an equal and opposite reaction. So during running, if your foot hits the ground in front of you, according to Newton, the ground pushes back. Essentially, you're putting on the brakes with every step. So shorten your stride and stop wasting your energy.

Most people take about 160 steps or so per minute. To check your stride rate, count all of your steps for 15 seconds, then multiply by four. If you're within 5 to 10 steps of 180, keep it up. If you're 10 or more steps per minute below that magic number, you should work to quicken your leg turnover. Doing that can be trickier than you might think; our next tip will address that. But once you master it, you will be a faster and more efficient runner.

FOCUS ON ARM POSITION AND SWING RATE

We run with our legs, of course, but that's not all we use when we run; our arms also play a very active role. Our arm swing counterbalances our leg swing, which helps us stay balanced as we move. Maintaining a good arm swing, then, is another element to having good overall running form.

The first key is to swing your arms from your shoulders; avoid twisting or rotating the body. Your torso should stay mostly still as your arms pump back and forth. This will reduce stress on your lower back and reduce the amount of energy it takes to move forward.

Second, keep your elbows bent relatively tightly, at about a 60-degree angle. If you run with your arms straighter, then you've created a long lever for your body to move. This wastes precious energy.

Third, make sure that you only swing forward and backward, and not across your body. Imagine that there's a wall coming straight out from your chest. If you tried to swing your arm across your body, it would smack into this wall. Use this image to help you straighten out your swing.

Finally, use your arms to increase your running cadence. If you try to speed up your stride by moving your legs faster, you'll find that it's harder to do than you might think. But since your leg turnover is tied to your arm swing, a quick and easy way to increase your leg turnover is to concentrate instead on swinging your arms faster. The best way to do this while maintaining good form is to focus on the backswing rather than the front swing. Aim to kick your elbows back faster and faster, and your legs will follow.

DON'T BOUNCE

It sounds like a simple idea, but it's often ignored: you get no credit in running for going up, only forward. Nevertheless, many runners lope like a gazelle, bouncing from step to step. That's good for gazelles, perhaps, but not so much for us. That's because everything that goes up must come down, and that drop puts excess stress on our bodies when we make impact with the ground. Exercise physiologists call this bouncing "vertical displacement," and we're going to aim to keep it to a minimum.

This is where a higher running cadence helps. When we take shorter, quicker steps, we naturally reduce our bounce because our time spent airborne is shorter, and so the arc of our flight is flatter.[17]

For some runners, bouncing is due not to low cadence, but to weakness in the quadriceps muscles. Recall that those muscles stabilize our legs on foot-strike. When they're too weak to do their job, they collapse and then rebound, creating that bounce effect. Strong quads mean less bounce. Keep your quads strong by doing squats or lunges as part of your regular cross-training strength program.

---

17 Interestingly, running faster also seems to mute our vertical displacement; you'll never see sprinters use a loping stride. That's one reason to work on getting faster—more on that in the next chapter.

MAINTAIN PROPER POSTURE

Proper posture in running is to be upright. In running lingo, this is referred to as running tall. Aim to keep your back straight; do not bend at the hips. If you run bent over, you'll put excess stress on your lower back, and you'll certainly feel the effects of that later.

Imagine that there is a rope attached to your chest that's pulling you upward toward a distant treetop. That pull will cause a slight forward lean, not just in your torso, but in your entire body. This lean will help create momentum, and it is why some coaches describe running as controlled forward falling.

If you can maintain proper form while running, you will not only reduce stress on your lower body, you will also set yourself up to run faster, as the forward falling will encourage you to take quick steps to catch yourself. Running tall will also enable you to breathe more deeply and easily.

RUNNING UP HILLS AND STAIRS

I haven't come across many people who like to do hill or stair workouts, but all runners should do them. Yes, they're hard, but they are great not just for building power and fitness, but also for improving form.

Running up hills and stairs works on improving explosive power but with relatively little impact. That's because your foot-strike occurs on a higher plane than you started—meaning that you are stepping *up*, so your foot is not dropping very far. At the same time, your leg muscles are working hard because they are not only propelling

THINK LIKE A **RUNNER**

you forward, but also lifting up your whole body, and doing it quickly. Use the down segment to rest and recover for the next repeat.

Beyond building better power and speed, running up hills and stairs improves form because it is impossible to overstride when going up. You simply cannot reach your leg as far in front of you as you might be used to doing while running on flat ground. For the same reason, you cannot heel-strike. You'll also find that you will naturally swing your arms more vigorously as you run up stairs or hills. That will prepare you for a quicker, sharper arm swing when you run on flat ground.

So, which is better: hills or stairs? Hills mimic a climb that you might find in a real race and can be incorporated into a regular run. You should look for a rise of about 100 meters, and if possible, find several options of varying steepness for slightly different workouts.

Stairs are more regular and regimented; after all, every hill can be different, but a flight of stairs is more or less the same everywhere. City parks often have good, long flights of stairs. If you have access to a building stairwell, you can do your stair workout in a controlled environment, a big benefit if you live somewhere that experiences cold winters.

If you run stairs, you also have two options: to run single steps, emphasizing speed and quick leg turnover, or double steps, emphasizing power.

RUNNING DRILLS

Drills are very different from exercises. While exercises aim to strengthen particular muscles, drills aim to reinforce motor patterns. For example, we would do push-ups to strengthen our chest, shoulders, and arms, but we would do backswing drills over and over to improve our tennis game.

Drills also differ from exercises in that they generally focus more on power than strength. Most people use these terms interchangeably, but for fitness professionals, they refer to very different things. *Strength* is the ability to move against resistance. *Power* involves how quickly you can move against resistance, which in exercise science is referred to as the rate of force production. It's the difference between doing a squat and jumping.

Running drills focus on each element of the running motion, exaggerating their movement to imprint that motor pattern on your brain. They also improve power since these drills are generally done quickly. The goal in doing drills is to provide a default setting for correct running form that your brain can automatically activate when running.

I recommend that you run drills at least once per week, although many runners do them two or three times. If you do speed-work on a track, it could be part of your warm-up. Each drill should be done on a 100-meter stretch of track or road. You can do one drill on the way out and another on the way back, or do a 50-meter out-and-back.

BUTT KICKS

This movement focuses on the follow-through of the push-off phase, when your hamstring muscles bend your knee. The drill is exactly what the name implies; kick your heels up as high as you can and as quickly as you can, with the imaginary goal of kicking yourself in the backside.

SOCCER KICKS

This movement focuses on the lift-off phase and aims to strengthen the hip flexor muscles on the front of your body. Keep your legs straight and knees locked out, then go up on your toes as you kick/run.

HIGH STEPS

This drill accentuates a strong knee lift during the lift-off phase. Aim to drive your knees as high as you can as you run down and back. Sometimes pairs of runners will do this drill as a team, with one runner standing still while they hold their hands palms down approximately waist-high. The other runner will quickly run in place, aiming to touch the palms with their knees. After 30 seconds, they switch positions. When doing this exercise, I like to imagine that I'm running on hot coals.

A SKIPS

Skipping improves takeoff and leg speed. It is similar to what we all did as kids, but with a few key differences. While we just swung our arms and bounced around as kids, when doing A skips, we want to keep our elbows tight and swing them strongly as we drive our opposite knee as high as we possibly can. They're usually done quickly without a lot of lift-off, but you can practice high-skipping as well to work more on power.

B SKIPS

Elite runners don't spend a lot of time with their feet on the ground; they aim to take quick, slapping steps, keeping "ground contact time" to a minimum. B skips are intended to emphasize the pull down and pawing off phases of running to keep this ground contact time to a minimum. They are similar to A skips but include an additional movement: at the highest point of knee lift, you'll swing your leg out as if you are kicking down a door, and then you'll pull it down sharply. So there are three parts to the movement: your knee goes up, your lower leg swings out, and your whole leg comes down. If you do these correctly, you'll hear a scraping sound as your foot hits the ground and paws off.

AGILITY DRILL/KARAOKE

Strictly speaking, this is not a drill as we've defined it because it doesn't mimic any part of the running motion. But it *is* a quick step movement that is designed to strengthen the outer hips and inner thighs—muscle groups that help maintain lateral stability during running. We do these by running sideways, crossing one leg in front of the other and then behind the other. Complete the drill by returning facing the same way, so that each leg now does the opposite movement. The image I have in my mind while doing these is of being in some big Broadway musical dance number. Silly, yes, but it helps.

———

You now have the tools to work with your body in order to run correctly. In the next chapter, we'll talk about running faster.

CHAPTER FIVE

SPEED: THE ALLURE OF RUNNING FAST

It didn't start out as a particularly special day. I put on my running clothes and shoes, had a light breakfast, and headed out to meet a group of friends for a run in the park. I expected to see most of the regulars; there was a core group of about a half-dozen of us who showed up regularly, and then there were a few more who would come out occasionally as their schedules and injuries allowed. We had been doing this for years.

It was, in many ways, the perfect training group for me. I was able to keep up, but most of the other runners were just a bit faster than me. I was always following the leader, although who would be the leader on a given day varied. That motivated and pushed me to run harder, which I liked. I believed that it made me a better runner.

On this morning, I met up with the group, and after a quick hello and some catching up, we set out on our run. We dropped down onto a trail, with the leader calling out the obstacles to avoid. "Rock!" "Roots!"

It was a cool morning; we were all dressed in tights and long-sleeve tops, but the path was dry and clear. The air smelled good, and I took a deep breath, feeling my chest expand. The cool air seemed to wake me up and energize me. I sped up and moved to the front of the pack.

This was a rare event for me, but not entirely unfamiliar. At one point or another we all took to the front and pushed the pace. Whoever felt best stayed up there and challenged everyone else to keep up.

My turn up front was usually brief, but not today. My legs felt like they were alive with energy, and the harder I ran, the better I felt. My breathing was strong and steady, and as my arms pumped, I focused intently on the trail in front of me.

Trail running requires concentration because every step must be instantly considered. You may be able to zone out while running down a smoothly paved street, but if you don't pay attention on a trail, you can suddenly find yourself face down in the dirt with a twisted ankle or worse.

Right then, I felt like a powerful machine. My concentration was laser-like, and my strides were smooth and strong.

My friend Adrian pulled up alongside me, expecting to pass me as would usually be the case. I wouldn't have minded it, but I had no intention of slowing down; the pace just felt so good.

After a mile, Adrian slipped back into the pack. Then it was Tai who pulled up alongside me. Tai is much taller than I am, and I often have difficulty matching his long strides. But not today. After a mile, he slipped back as well.

We ran on. I heard the breathing getting raspy and a bit ragged behind me. Midway through the run someone called out, "Okay, Jeff, you win!" I laughed and shrugged my shoulders.

"Guys, I don't know what's going on today," I said, honestly, laughing.

Then it was over. We were back to our starting spot, steam rising off our bodies as we gasped for air and moved around, cooling down.

I knew that I would always remember that day, and indeed, years later, it's still as vivid to me as the moment it happened. It is near the top of my lifetime list of best running experiences. I had relished that wild feeling, when my body felt like it had harnessed some great power and had channeled it into pure motion. I had asked my legs to push harder, and miraculously, unbelievably, they did. I wanted to run faster, and faster still, to the very end of the trail.

I had tapped into something primal, something almost beyond words, something that felt close to immortality. I had experienced the thrill of pushing my body to its limit, and I basked in the afterglow of wobbly legs and exhausted elation.

I'd experienced speed.

DEFINING SPEED

The term "speed" dates back to the Middle Ages, appearing with slight variations in Old English (spede or spowan) to Old High German (spout), Old Saxon (spodian), and Dutch (spoed). The term meant to succeed or prosper. It was only later that the word evolved to reflect velocity, itself defined as the rate of the distance traveled by an object to the time required to travel that distance—miles per hour, feet per second. Eventually, the reference to success faded, and the word came to mean swiftness itself.

Reducing the meaning of speed to an intersection of time and distance, however, misses a larger meaning of the word. Speed is not just an objective measurement based on recorded data. It is a subjective experience, a sensation, an experience.

Speed is one of the elemental urges wired into our DNA. From the moment we begin to crawl, to when we learn to walk and run, we are driven to go faster. Perhaps it's a vestigial reminder of our days in the jungle or open plains, when failure to move swiftly could have meant death, whether from a predator or from the failure to catch prey.

Or maybe it was one of the ways our ancestors ensured their survival. If you were able to run faster, you might rise higher in the clan's hierarchy and win the most appealing mate, perpetuating your lineage.

Luckily, our ascendancy to the top of the food chain didn't depend on foot speed alone. But even as our big brains and opposable thumbs gave us an evolutionary advantage, the thrill of speed remained. No matter how our own individual running speeds match up against other animals or our peers, there are few physical sensations that match the joy of running fast. Everything else—finish lines, victories, world records—is a result of that fact, not a cause of it.

We can only guess at why we run, but what we do know, intuitively, is that running fast feels right. It feels good. It can feel great.

Let's look at what fast really means. The average running speed of humans for relatively short distances is between 13 and 20 miles per hour, and between 5 and 13 miles per hour over long distances. The current world record for the 100-meter distance is 9.58 seconds, set by Usain Bolt in 2009, which translates to 23.4 miles per hour. For even shorter distances, humans can go as fast as 28 miles per hour. For the marathon, the current record is 2:00:35, set by Kelvin Kiptum in 2023,[18] which translates into about 13 miles per hour.

Those records sound crazy fast to most of us, but compared to other fleet-footed animals, these speeds aren't particularly impressive. The fastest land animal, the cheetah, has been recorded as hitting 70 to 75 miles per hour over 500 meters (roughly 1,600 feet). The American quarter horse, meanwhile, can hit 55 miles per hour in full gallop, and even your house cat can race away from your broken lamp at about 30 miles per hour.

For much of my running career, I've been an above-average runner, but I'm not particularly gifted. I've qualified for the Boston Marathon, and I used to routinely place in the top half of the pack in my races, often in the top 10 to 25 percent of the field. But if you consider how much time, effort, and thought I've put into running, you'd have to conclude that my achievements are modest at best. There's a world of difference between

---

18 Kelvin Kiptum tragically died in a car accident in his homeland of Kenya on February 11, 2024.

finishing in the top 10 percent of runners in a race and finishing in the top 10. I'm clearly not an elite runner.

But still, I revel in the speed that I do have, and I love to think back on my fastest moments, like that one morning running in the woods with my friends. Lately I've begun to wonder a bit more deeply about this. There is a German word, I was once told, that essentially means enjoying that which you can do well. All of us have evolved to run, and to run fast, even if that's a relative term.

As thinking runners, our task is to solve this Gordian knot that is running and figure out the best way to get better at it. That includes working to get faster.

To some degree, this will happen naturally without any special effort. As we get more fit and more efficient as runners, our speed will naturally improve, even if we don't do anything in particular to bring about that result. But at some point your speed will top out, and you won't get any faster with your regular training routine.

This is a crossroads of sorts. At this point, you can just continue running as you have been. You will still get all the physical, mental, and emotional benefits of running. But if you want to continue to get faster, you will have to start training specifically for that. To run fast, you have to practice fast running.

TRAINING FOR SPEED

The first kind of speed that we all experience—what we can call playground speed—is a kind of immature speed. By that I mean that it lacks structure and discipline. To a young child playing with friends in the schoolyard, there is basically one speed to running: you go as fast as you can until you drop.

Adult speed, or athletic speed, is something else. Speed is like a car with manual transmission; to use it properly, you have to know what gear to engage and when to engage it. To do that, whether driving or running, requires practice and discipline. The key to training for speed, then, is to know how fast to run, for what distance, and how many times.

Suddenly, speed is not just a matter of raw power; it's a mental challenge.

It wasn't always this way. Speed-work, as we know it now, is a fairly modern invention, dating back only a bit over a century. Before that, endurance athletes simply ran or walked long distances. It wasn't until the early 1900s that the concept of interval training was invented.

INTERVAL TRAINING

Interval training, the practice of running short, fast distances repeatedly, with a slow recovery run in between each, was first widely introduced by a Finnish coach, Lauri Pihkala, who trained, among others, the great Olympic champion Paavo Nurmi. In a 1918 letter to Nurmi, Coach Pihkala gave detailed instructions for a speed session, including paces for different repeated short runs, to end with a series of sprints.

The thinking behind this new approach was that an athlete could run faster for several short distances than they could run for one long distance, and that the result of these short, repeated efforts would be an increase in speed that was unattainable with longer, slower runs.

With this insight, modern training was born.

The 1930s saw the introduction of another kind of training: fartlek intervals. Meaning "speed-play," this form of training developed in Sweden and involved incorporating repeated unstructured bursts of fast running during a longer run. This kind of running was intuitive and spontaneous; you would decide to pick up your pace for a given distance as you felt the urge. This brought running back around to the school-yard—think, "From here to the light post, as fast as you can; go!"—but it still involved the concept of repeats and recoveries. This method was popular and effective in the years before the outbreak of World War II.

During this period, the German coach Woldemar Gerschler refined interval training by linking efforts and recovery with heart rates. His insight was that fitness and improvement were governed by the recovery period; improvements in intensity and speed were to be based on how long it took for an athlete's heart rate to recover after hard efforts. Gerschler coached that the training load should become more challenging as the recovery periods decreased; as his athletes became faster and more fit, he would make their workouts harder.

In the early postwar period, the great Czech Olympian Emil Zátopek revolutionized speed-work with his long, brutal sprint workouts. He would do workouts that no one else had dared to even consider, pushing his body to do up to 40 sprints in a workout, interspersed with short recovery runs. In his simple and eminently quotable words, he defended his training methods.

When I was young, I was too slow. I thought I must learn to run fast by practicing to run fast, so I ran 100 meters fast 20 times. Then I came back, slow, slow, slow. People said, 'Emil,

you are crazy. You are training like a sprinter.' Why should
I practice running slow? I already know how to run slow. I
want to learn to run fast.[19]

Fast is what he got. For his efforts, Zátopek, aka the Czech Locomotive, won one silver and four gold medals in the 1948 and 1952 Olympics in the 5K, the 10K, and the marathon.

Modern science has refined speed-work by using objective guideposts rather than simple intuition. Coaches talk about lactate thresholds, heart rate zones, and anaerobic thresholds— the points at which the body reaches the limit of its aerobic capacity and shifts into another mode of fueling. Workouts are now designed to push athletes to the edge of these limits week after week, triggering improvements that lead to even harder workouts.

GET COMFORTABLE WITH DISCOMFORT

If this is all starting to sound a bit too intense for you, don't worry. You don't need to use a heart rate monitor or have your blood analyzed to become a faster runner. The hardest part about becoming a faster runner is not to learn to master the science of running; it's about learning to master your own aversion to discomfort.

Running fast hurts. Anyone who tells you otherwise is sugarcoating the truth. The key to becoming a faster runner is to accept the pain and learn to handle it.

Now, before you throw this book across the room, let me be clear: I'm not talking about injury-level pain, the kind that tells you that you've just strained your Achilles tendon or torn

---

19 Lee Glandorf, "When It Hurts, Go Faster," *Tracksmith Journal*, https://www.tracksmith.com/journal/article/when-it-hurts-go-faster.

your ACL. I'm talking extreme discomfort. Think about your pleasant Sunday morning long run, when your mind wanders or you chat with your running friend, and you notice the buds that have suddenly appeared on the trees that you pass.

Speed-work is nothing like that. Instead of noticing more, you notice less. Your world shrinks until it is focused only on maintaining your pace. You breathe and lock your eyes on the stretch of road or track in front of you. You have no extra breath to talk, and there is nothing to say even if you could. If you have a mantra, you repeat it in your head over and over. "Keep it going, almost there, left right left right left right!" If you are running with others, you fight to maintain your place in the pack, or to even move up a spot or two.

None of this is comfortable. Nonetheless, you may enjoy it. Or you may not. But that's not the point. You are not doing this to have fun. You are doing this to improve your running, to be faster. When you want to have a good time, go for a nice long weekend run. But when you head out for your speed session, you need to get your mind in the right place. Focus on what you are about to do, what it will feel like, and how good it will feel to get through the workout. Think about how these workouts will stack up, like gold in the bank, and how much you will enjoy being rich in speed.

TO TRACK OR NOT TO TRACK?

Speed sessions are typically held on a regulation track, and there's a reason for that. Within the controlled confines of your local high school or rec center track, distractions and obstacles that could hinder your performance have been eliminated. There are no potholes, red lights, pedestrians, or stray dogs. There is also no guesswork; the distance is precisely measured, which means that every effort can be compared to every other similar effort, and progress can be effectively gauged.

The benefit of this approach is even greater than it might at first appear. With honest, reliable data available to you about your speed at different distances, you can begin to associate effort levels with particular speeds. After running quarter-mile, half-mile, and one-mile intervals on the track, and recording your times for each repeat, you will develop a familiarity with the discomfort that each one produces. Here's the important part: this works both ways. So when you run, and you reach a certain level of discomfort, you can be pretty sure that you've hit that same speed.

This is one of the main benefits of running on the track: the internalization of the link between running efforts and speed. Having an intuitive sense of how fast you're going gives you the opportunity to control your speed by feel alone, which is crucial to being a purposeful runner. Is your goal to be able to run an 8-minute mile in training? It would help you immensely if you knew what that felt like.

But can the benefits of speed-work be achieved off the track? Absolutely. You can do your sessions on the treadmill, which provides the added bonus of forcing you to run the speed that you set it for. Rather than checking your watch to make sure that you're hitting your goals, you are guaranteed success simply by keeping up with the spinning tread. Sure, it's not much fun to keep having to adjust the speed control, and there is a short lag time until the treadmill gets up to speed, but overall, this works.

If you're considering this option, here's a little tip: if you find yourself losing track of how many laps you've done, use my penny method. Simply line up on the left side of the monitor a penny for each repeat that you plan to do, and move a penny to the right or toss it to the floor after you've completed each planned repeat. When you're out of pennies, your workout is over.

And, of course, there are the roads. You may not get the same precision here as you would on the track or on the treadmill, but you can still get the job done. You can measure distances as closely as possible to the planned workout, or you can just plan to run at a certain effort level for a precise amount of time, whatever the distance ends up being. Whatever you choose to do, remember that running repeats of any kind will make you faster, even if they are not measured with total accuracy.

BE DISCIPLINED

There's a catch to this, however. To be a good runner, you need to be disciplined. That doesn't always mean that every fast run should be run as fast as you can go, or that the more difficult a workout feels, the better it must be for you. Being a good runner means matching your effort level to that workout's specific goals. Success means that you have done exactly that; nothing less and nothing more.

This is harder to comply with than you might think, but it's crucial. We develop different speeds so that we can deploy them in different settings. When we run an appropriately challenging speed for a specified distance, we trigger a specific adaptation.

For endurance runners, this almost always involves improving our aerobic capacity and pushing against the boundaries of our lactate threshold. If we push past that limit, we stop working in the aerobic zone. Instead, we begin to work anaerobically, fueling ourselves from a different pathway, training our bodies in a different mode. Simply put, we become endurance athletes who are instead training like sprinters. That would make it the wrong workout for the sport we're in.

The key, then, is to have the right mindset. It's fine to be competitive with the other athletes around you during the workout, but never forget that your workout is yours alone; you are not there to run their workouts. So if you are supposed to run your 800-meter repeats at a 5K race pace—a common speed session goal— do not sprint out ahead at a pace much faster than your best 5K time. Or if the repeat is supposed to feel like an 8 out of 10 effort, don't push so hard that you're gasping at a 9.5 out of 10 level. Even if you complete the workout, and even if you don't end up suffering an injury from it, this is not a sustainable, safe, or effective way to train.

Again, remember our mantra: be smarter than you are brave. Just because you can will yourself through that kind of brutality doesn't make it a good idea to do so.

PLANNING TO RUN SPEED

Once you commit to doing speed-work, the issue of logistics inevitably arises. Basic questions need to be answered. There are no set rules on this, but there does seem to be a consensus among coaches about how to incorporate these workouts into your routine.

Plan to do speed-work once a week. No more, no less. Remember: any increase in training stimulus introduces a risk of injury. We push a little harder in order to improve our fitness, but as you recall, if we push too hard, we can get hurt. A good, well-thought-out training program minimizes the risk of injury while triggering improvement by moderating the stimulus. Doing speed-work once per week generally fits the bill. Doing it more often than that might prove to be just a bit too much. Can you handle it anyway? Maybe, but why risk it for minimal to nonexistent additional gain? Be smart.

Decide on a program. You can connect with a coach or a local training program, or you can find speed progressions online. I'll recommend a few on the next page. There is science to this, but everyone is a little different and responds to training in slightly different ways. There are many different types of programs that might bring you success, so you shouldn't feel like you need to find the one true program. Do the one that fits you best at the time. Done correctly, any speed-work program will bring gains.

Decide with whom to run. Speed-work is taxing not just physically, but mentally as well—you've probably picked up on that by this point. That's why many runners choose to do their speed workouts in groups, where they can feed off the group energy, find hidden reserves after being encouraged by their peers, and enjoy the afterglow of a job well done in the company of comrades. It's certainly possible to do these workouts alone, but why make a hard thing harder than it needs to be? Misery loves company. This old phrase applies here in spades. Make use of your friends.

Decide on your workouts. If you are working with a coach, following a program, or running with a club, this will be decided for you—you just need to follow the workouts that you're given.

If you're training on your own, however, you need to decide on your own workouts. This can seem daunting. There are many workouts and progressions to follow, and this could also be the subject of an entire book. Don't let yourself get lost in the weeds on this, however. In other words, don't overthink this. If you pick a few good workouts and do them to the best of your ability once a week, you will get results. Here are my three favorites:

- **800-meter repeats.** Run anywhere from 6 to 10 of these, with a 400-meter easy recovery lap between each. Your pace should be moderately hard, about equal to your 5K race pace. This is the meat and potatoes of speed-work—an all-purpose workout that brings benefits for a wide range of distances, from the 5K to the marathon.
- **1-mile repeats.** Run between 3 and 6 of these, with a 400-meter easy recovery. Your pace should be about equal to your 10K race pace. These are harder, physically and mentally, than running the shorter distances. I find them to be most appropriate in training for longer races, like the half-marathon and the marathon.

- **100-meter sprints.** Run from 10 to 20 of these, with a very short 10-second recovery between each. These are high intensity, so run at a very hard level. This is a very hard workout, but it goes by quickly. Make sure that you're fully warmed up beforehand.

If you plan your own speed workouts, keep in mind that the total volume should generally be less than you do for your long runs, or even for your training runs. Again, this is about moderating risk: you can run far, and you can run fast, but each will raise the risk of injury just a little bit, and running both far and fast will raise the risk much higher.

For this reason, you will see that most speed-work sessions call for a total of 3 to 5 miles of speed, with a few more easy miles for the warm-up, recovery laps, and cool-down. This limit seems to be a coach's rule of thumb, and as with most rules of thumb, it may not be 100 percent scientifically proven. But it's based on common experience and collective wisdom and will probably serve you well.

AND NOW WHAT?

My friend Jeff S. is an enigma to me. He's a cyclist, but that's not what interests me in particular. It's his training routine. Jeff follows a strict program, logging his miles, workouts, and paces carefully over the year. He monitors his speed, power, and distance not just from week to week and month to month, but from year to year, and spends time analyzing the data, tinkering with the workouts, and trying out new ideas. Jeff is what you would call performance oriented.

But here's the thing: Jeff doesn't train hard in order to perform well on race day, because there is no race day for him.

As far as I know, he has never participated in an organized cycling event, and he has no interest in ever doing so.

I find this to be unusual and more than a little intriguing. Most athletes I know either train moderately for health and enjoyment, or train for performance on event day, but I'd never before met anyone who worked through a challenging and difficult training program without having a race on their calendar.

What is Jeff thinking?

The answer, I believe, is that he is motivated by the pure enjoyment of working hard for a goal he has set for himself, with the objective of achieving that goal on his own terms, for his private sense of accomplishment. There will be no cheering crowds or finisher medals for Jeff, but he has no need for that. What does all that matter anyway? He'll know what he's achieved, and that's enough. He might share his accomplishments with the friends he trains with, like me, and that will be more meaningful than the applause of strangers because these cycling buddies have been there for much of his training and should share in his sense of achievement.

But Jeff doesn't rest on his laurels for too long. Each season brings a new opportunity to test training theories and to see if he can once again seize the brass ring.

That's my friend Jeff S., but that isn't me. While I can appreciate his perspective, admire his determination and work ethic, and applaud his accomplishment, I need that event on my race calendar to get me motivated.

In the next chapter we'll talk more deeply about the excitement of putting all the hard work to the test. We'll talk about racing.

CHAPTER SIX

RACING

I've been told that in parts of Texas they tell a joke about something called a post turtle. This is an ordinary turtle that somehow finds itself sitting on top of a fence post. From that vantage point, the turtle can think only of two things: how the heck did I get up here, and how the heck can I get down?

I thought of that story a few years ago when, to my great surprise, I found myself in third place in a local 5K road race. Granted, it wasn't the NYC Marathon, where there might be 47,000 other runners. There were perhaps 50 or 60 other racers, and no one, as far as I knew, had traveled more than a half hour or so to get from their home to the race start. But still, there I was, ahead of all but two of them.

In over two decades of racing, I've had some special moments, but I've only very rarely been close to winning an award. I've had dreams of leading the pack to the finish line, however. In some of these dreams, I've gotten lost and managed to lose the race, but as my friends have told me, these dreams aren't really about running. Maybe not. In any case, my dresser top still remains glaringly uncluttered by any trophies or plaques.

All of which left me surprised and even amused that I found myself in a race with only two people in front of me.

The race hadn't started out as anything special. It was run on an out-and-back course through a local park, starting with a short flat section, followed by a long, steep downhill, more flat running to the turnaround, and then a hard climb back up that hill and on to the finish line.

I knew the course well, since I had trained on it regularly, and had even raced the same course a few months earlier. But there was nothing about the way I had run that road previously, or by the way that I felt that morning, that would lead me to believe that this would be a different kind of day.

I began the race with a friend, and though we never discussed it, I assumed we'd run together for most, or all, of the race. We chatted for a bit, but when we turned left and began the descent down the big hill, I surged ahead. I wasn't making any kind of strategic move; I was only taking advantage of all that downhill by doing a controlled fall. The road would level out, and I assumed that soon after I'd find myself somewhere deep in the pack.

Except that I didn't. Instead, I came off the hill feeling strong, and I surged ahead, enjoying the moment. I passed a few people, and then a few more. I knew who the leader was; I had spotted him before the race began as looking like someone who could run fast, and sure enough, he ran away from the rest of us as soon as the race started.

But in front of me now, I could only see one other person. Ahead of him there was just open road. Slowly I began to realize that he might very well be in second place. Which meant, of course, that I was third.

Holy cow!

Around the time that thought crossed my mind, the first-place runner blew past us going the opposite way, back toward the hill that we had just descended. There would be no catching him. But as I looked down the road, I realized that this guy right in front of me, well, *he* was catchable. If I could pull off that feat, I'd be in *second* place.

Holy cow again!

The question for me now was how to go about it. For the first time in all my years of racing, I needed to come up with a plan, a strategy for beating this one guy on whom I had set my sights.

I approached the problem like a hunter, methodically and patiently. I decided to pull near to him before the turnaround, and when we took the turn and momentarily lost our rhythm, I would put on a quick burst of speed to open a gap. The suddenness of my move would, I hoped, catch him by surprise. Then I would use the uphill, which I knew so well, to pull away and drop him for good.

With my plan in mind, I began to surge ahead to draw even with my rival. As I came alongside him, I gave him a quick, "Hey, how ya doing?" delivered in the most calm, controlled voice I could muster. I hoped that when he heard my voice, he would think that I was running well below my capacity. I wanted him to believe that his top speed was just an easy pace for me, and that if he were to push me, I would punish him by accelerating into a pace that he could never match.

In other words, I tried to lie to him.

Shockingly, my plan seemed to work. We rounded the turn-around cones and I leapt ahead, deftly switching places with him. It was such an unlikely position for me to be in that I felt like laughing. I was that post turtle, except that I wasn't really looking to get down. I was gonna ride this thing out to the end and see where it could take me.

I held my place as we passed the two-mile mark, and looked ahead toward an upcoming sharp right turn and the hill that would immediately follow. If I pulled ahead just a bit more, I would be out of my rival's view for a few moments after I made that turn. A quick, strong move at the base of the hill could put me far enough up the hill to dash any hope he had of catching me. It would hurt, but if I could do it, I felt certain that second place would be mine.

I made the turn and jumped ahead, hoping that my plan wouldn't leave me gasping for air and reduced to a walk as my competitor, running a smarter and more patient race, blazed past.

I gritted my teeth and took the discomfort, and when I looked over my shoulder, the gap between me and the other guy had doubled. Even as I slowed down on the hill, he dropped even farther back. He had given up. He didn't believe catching me was possible, so he wasn't willing to suffer by trying. My little plan had worked.

I came off the hill and turned right, located the finish line in my sights, and began my final drive. I looked over my shoulder one more time. I was all alone. I could have slowed down a bit then, but I felt the need to give it all I had as I drove on to the end.

I crossed the finish line gasping. When the awards ceremony was held, I stepped forward to claim my reward—a $25 gift card to a local running store—and to pose for a photograph with the first and third place runners. I felt like royalty.

At almost the same time that I was racing, another 5K was taking place a few miles away. A good friend of mine was competing in that race, and as soon as mine was over, I called to see how he did. He, too, had taken second place, except that his finishing time was several *minutes* faster than mine. In his race, I might not even have finished in the top 20.

I didn't care. In my race, I was the second-best runner there. I replayed every step of the race in my mind countless times over the following weeks, and every time I did so, I realized one thing: racing is *fun*. I mean *really* fun. Not just because I did well, but also because I had challenged myself, and in giving it my all, I felt a sense of accomplishment that I hardly ever get just from training. Running changed my life, but racing brought me to a different world entirely.

You're probably expecting me now to lay out all the reasons why you should consider racing. That would be the obvious move, so let's go in a different direction. Let's start out with the reasons why you should *not* race.

THE DRAWBACKS OF RACING

IT CAN BE EXPENSIVE

When I ran my first marathon decades ago, the entrance fee was $15. Times have changed. It's common now to pay ten times that or more to register for a marathon, and to pay $50 or more to participate even in short races like the 5K. I do understand that expenses have gone up for the race organizers, especially the cost of providing necessary police to maintain road closures.

Nevertheless, if you plan to race on a regular basis, registration can become a big budget item.

Add on top of this the cost of travel and accommodation. In all likelihood, there are many races that are held right in your hometown, from the Thanksgiving Turkey Trot, to the Fourth of July Firecracker, to the Christmas Jingle Bell run. But if you feel the urge to participate in a big out-of-town race, like the Chicago Marathon or the Boston Marathon, you have to add in transportation and hotel expenses. I once took a shot at estimating the amount of money I've spent over the years on pursuing my hobby, and it was staggering. I'm not saying that I regret it—far from it—but it is something to consider.

IT CAN BE A LOGISTICAL HASSLE

The wonderful thing about the sport of running is that your experience can start as soon as you head out your front door. There is no need to reserve court time or to travel to an arena. Just put on your shoes and go.

That is, unless you want to race. If you're racing locally, then all you have to do is figure out how to get back and forth from the start. Maybe you can carpool with friends, or take public transportation, or arrange to get dropped off or picked up by a loved one or even a taxi service. There's a hassle factor here, but it's manageable.

But maybe you want to run a big race in another city. That takes planning. In addition to travel and lodging, you must decide on the clothing and gear that you'll bring. Both the fall and spring race seasons straddle the transition between warm and cold weather, often making race day temperatures unpredictable. That means you will probably need to bring a range of clothing and gear to handle whatever weather you may encounter.

The nightmare scenario is that the weather will suddenly change dramatically, leaving you unprepared. I was in Delaware in December years ago, getting ready for a marathon the following morning, when I found out that an arctic blast was descending overnight, dropping the temperatures more than 30 degrees below normal. It was winter, but I was unprepared for that sudden change. I improvised by wearing sweatpants over my running tights and socks over my gloves. On the course, I saw other runners had ice on their hats; their sweat had frozen solid. I kept running out of fear of freezing if I stopped, and I swore that I would never again come to a race unprepared for every possibility. But, boy, that can quickly fill luggage to the breaking point.

IT CAN BE AN ECOLOGICAL NIGHTMARE

All you need to do to see the impact of racing on the environment is to sign up to be a finish line volunteer. When all the participants have crossed the finish line and gone home, there are hundreds or thousands of paper cups, bottles, and food wrappers that need to be disposed of. There will even be discarded clothes and other gear lying around. That all adds up to a lot of space in a landfill.

Race directors are not unmindful about this. There has been a big effort over the past decade to make most of the advertisements and promotional materials given to racers virtual so that there is less paper waste, and discarded clothing is usually collected and donated. Many races have also eliminated cups and instead require racers to bring their own water bottles for refill at aid stations. Still, the environmental impact of the many hundreds of races that are held across the nation every year is substantial.

IT'S ALL A BIT ARTIFICIAL

By definition, a race is a competition, but the vast majority of runners in any given race have no chance of finishing in the top 10, let alone winning, and they know this. So why race? If you want to run a 5K, a 10K, or even a marathon, then just head out the door and do it. You don't have to pay anyone for that privilege.

I'm reminded of a friend of mine, Cathy F., who trained to run her first marathon. She decided to make her last long training run the full marathon distance, and after successfully completing that run, she decided not to do the race. When she told me this, I was confused.

"But you trained for it," I said to her, "and now you're completely ready. All that's left is for you to do the same thing on race day, and you'll have completed a marathon."

"But I *have* completed a marathon," Cathy replied.

I had to grudgingly admit the logic of what she'd said. If her goal was to prove to herself that she could complete the marathon distance, then she'd already achieved that goal. What more would she get by running that distance again on race day? A medal that she'd put in a drawer? A T-shirt that she might never wear? The cheers of strangers? She'd decided that all of that was beside the point. Much like Shakespeare's Hamlet, she had decided that "the readiness is all." I wanted to contradict her, but I had to admit that there was something pure and true in her point of view.

This can lead us to ponder a bigger question: What is a race? You run from point to point, but in fact there's nothing particularly special or magical about any distance. Even the 26.2 miles that constitute the marathon, perhaps the most storied of all races, is arbitrary. A quote from the famous jurist Oliver Wendell Holmes Jr., written over a century ago, applies here: "A page of history is worth a volume of logic."[20]

ORIGINS OF THE MARATHON

The story is that in 490 B.C. the Athenians lined up against the Persians on the Plains of Marathon, badly outnumbered and facing likely defeat. Miraculously, they triumphed—this much is true. Then, legend has it, the courier Pheidippides raced the roughly 25 miles from the battle site back to Athens to pass along the good news to the women, children, and old men who were waiting anxiously to hear their fate. "Nike!" he allegedly cried out—"We are victorious!" And then, supposedly, he died.

Enamored with this story, the organizers of the modern Olympic Games decided to make the 25-mile race an event to be called the "marathon," after the site of that ancient battle. This was especially appropriate, since those games were to be held in Athens. In 1908 the games were held in London, and the race was extended to 26.2 miles in deference to the British royal family so that they could see the finish line from the royal box.

---

20 New York Trust Co. v. Eisner, 256 U.S. 345 (1921).

To this, we must now admit that the finishing order is arbitrary as well. As admitted at the beginning of this chapter, my glorious second-place finish in that local 5K was achieved not just because I ran a strong, smart race, but because other much faster runners didn't happen to show up. If a thousand other faster runners had been there, I would not even have been in the top 1,000. That's true even if I had managed to run my fastest 5K ever. So while I'm proud of that effort, and I can brag about that second place finish to my running friends and to you, I know that it is due as much to luck as to effort.

IT ISN'T NEEDED TO STAY HEALTHY

You certainly don't need to race to get all the health benefits of running. In fact, I am saddened at the thought that some race participants have worked to achieve their bucket list dream of finishing a race, only to return to a sedentary lifestyle after they've hit their goal. It would have been much better for their health for them to have skipped the race and instead kept up with a steady training routine.

In fact, racing can actually be bad for you. If you are at a higher risk for certain types of heart attacks, as even some accomplished runners are, then racing can be a high-risk activity for you.[21] There's even some evidence that very long distance racing can lead to scarring in the heart and elevated levels of certain kinds of plaque.[22]

---

21 Bethany Rolfe Witham and Keven Babbitt, "Cardiovascular Risks in Long Distance Runners," *Journal of Christian Nursing* 34, no. 2 (April/June 2017): 97–101.

22 Omar Jafar et al., "Assessment of Coronary Atherosclerosis Using Calcium Scores in Short- and Long-Distance Runners," *Mayo Clinic Proceedings: Innovations, Quality & Outcomes* 3, no. 2 (June 2019): 116–21.

So, if racing is an expensive hassle that pollutes and is based on arbitrary distances, and your placement at the finish line is pure chance, and it may not even be all that great for you, what's the point? Why race?

THE BENEFITS OF RACING

Now I get to make the case for racing. Despite the drawbacks we just discussed, racing adds things to my life that outweigh all the negatives.

IT CREATES ORDER AND STRUCTURE

Having a race on my calendar creates order in the chaos of my life. Once I have that deadline looming on my horizon, I force myself to stick to a routine that will prepare me for the race. My days and weeks become structured, and I become motivated to push myself harder than I would had I not committed myself to that event. Letting my friends and family know that I'm planning to do a race only adds more motivation to get my act together, since I would hate to disappoint their expectations of me on race day.

You may respond to this by pointing out that my logic on this is circular—I race so that I'll train, and I train so that I'll be able to race. Well, you're probably right, but so what? It works, at least for me. It gets me out of bed and on the roads on cold mornings when I'd rather sleep in. It gets me to do long runs, hill repeats, and speed-work when I'd rather take it easy, and getting out there makes me healthier and happier.

I should be able to do all that hard training without registering for a race, just like my cycling friend Jeff S., but I know me, and I know that I won't. Racing is the lever and the rope to push and pull and prod me into getting the best out of myself in a way that I could never do all on my own. I know there are many, many other people for whom racing has this same effect.

IT ALLOWS YOU TO EXPLORE NEW PLACES

There's no better way to see a new place than by running through it, and there is no better way to run through it than in a race. Most races, especially marathons, are designed to show off the highlights of the city, so a race is really a guided tour, with cheerleaders and support along the way and a medal at the end. No need to plan out the route or worry about traffic. It's all taken care of. What's not to like?

Some of the best moments of my life have occurred when I was running races in new places. I've been fortunate enough to have had the opportunity to race past the pyramids in Cairo, through the Brandenburg Gate in Berlin, in the shadow of Mount Everest in India, down the Avenue des Champs-Élysées in Paris, over the Tower Bridge in London, and on the Pacific Coast Highway in California. I loved every sweaty minute of it.

IT MAKES ME A BETTER PERSON

Yes, racing may be arbitrary, at least in the way we just talked about it, and yes, you don't need to race to get all the health benefits of running. But racing is ultimately not about time or distance or health. It's about proving to ourselves that we can overcome our doubts and our fears of failure and become something better than we thought we were. If we can do that on race day, what else might we be able to achieve at home, at work, and in life?

If there is really one great thing about racing, at least for me, it's exactly that. As Shakespeare wrote in *Julius Caesar*, "Bid me run, and I will strive with things impossible."[23]

Against that, all the other complaints about racing seem to melt away. Sure, it costs money, but we all spend money on things that give us far less joy. If I need to budget for a race and give up some other things, so be it.

Yes, race day can be a hassle, but *life* is a hassle. Figure it out and make it happen.

Yes, racing has a carbon footprint, but that footprint has been reduced, and we can encourage race directors to do an even better job at that.

IT MAKES ME PART OF A COMMUNITY

If nothing I've said so far in support of racing has lit a fire beneath you, consider this: racing is not just about targeting a day on your calendar to do your best; it's also about connecting with the running community at large and making a public declaration about ourselves and our values.

When we gather in our tens of thousands on race day in Boston, London, Chicago, or New York City, we become an example for ourselves and others of determination and self-sufficiency.

When I raced in the Indian Himalayas, I learned the meaning of the greeting "Namaste," which, I was told, means "the light within me recognizes the light within you." It is a beautiful concept, reflecting a model of respect for one's self and for all people; it is a declaration of our common humanity and of the sacredness of life.

---

23 *Julius Caesar*, Act 2 Scene 1.

This, I believe, is the same feeling that my fellow racers and I share at the starting line. Even if none of us think of it in those exact words, our actions show it, as we make room for each other and wish each other good luck. It's shown during the race when we offer each other encouragement and even hand off water and supplies to each other. It's shown after the race when we racers—strangers, but yet somehow not really complete strangers anymore—congratulate each other, fist bump, high-five, and, sometimes, even hug and cry.

If it's true that all the world's a stage, then racing is the triumph of drama over tragedy, when hope and faith are rewarded, when we can see what can be accomplished by dreaming people who manage to make those dreams come true. Racing—not just running, but *racing*—brings the beautiful realization that there are many, many other people who share this same dream. And if this can be done in running, can it not also be done everywhere, with all of our problems?

Am I saying that racing can help save the world? Well, maybe I am.

After I wrote those last words, I read them out loud to my wife. I expected her to swoon with emotion. Instead, there was silence.

"Well," I prompted. "What do you think?"

"Well, you certainly do sound passionate," she deadpanned.

Pause.

"Um, did I oversell it a bit?"

Pause.

"Yeah, maybe."

So, OK, maybe racing won't save the world. But I think it can certainly help make our lives better, and I think you should give it a chance.

GETTING READY TO RACE

Once you've made the decision to race, there's work to be done. First, you need to decide the distance that you want to race, where you want to race, and when you want to race. Then you will have to create a training schedule and a race plan.

All of this can seem overwhelming to a new racer, but like all things in life, and as with running in particular, it will all be easier if we take it step by step.

CHOOSING A RACE DISTANCE AND LOCATION

There are many factors that figure into deciding on a race distance, but your overriding consideration should be picking a distance that you feel that you will be prepared to race. Think about the training that you have already done and the training that you consider reasonable going forward. If your runs have been no farther than a few miles at a time, then a short race may be the one for you. But if you've become comfortable with longer runs, then you may want to be more ambitious.

In general, I recommend that you approach racing conservatively. You can start with a 5K and work your way up to longer distances as you get more training and racing under your belt and mature as a runner, both physically and emotionally. If you start more aggressively, you may risk having a bad experience that will discourage you from racing, or worse, leave you injured. Remember: there is no rush to this.

Having said that, I now have a confession to make: my very first race of any kind was a marathon. While I don't recommend that for most people, it made sense for me.

This was my thinking. I had built up my training, and I was already doing around 40 miles per week, with long runs of around 10 miles. I realized that while I was developing into a decent runner, I was no speedster. My chances of being near the top finishers in a 5K race were slim to none. Meanwhile, the 5K distance itself didn't seem challenging because I routinely had training runs that were two or three times that distance. So, I thought, if I wasn't going to be competitive in the race, and simply finishing wasn't going to feel like much of an accomplishment, then this wasn't the race for me.

That's where the marathon came in. First, it captured my imagination because it was such a famous and historic distance. I immediately fell prey to the marathon mystique.

But the attraction was greater than that. The marathon seemed to me to be such a daunting distance—more than double the farthest distance that I had yet run. Instead of scaring me off, however, this became the race's main attraction for me. My speed would not be a factor; simply finishing the race would be the goal. Because I had doubts (fears, actually) about my ability to run it, I knew that I would be diligent in my preparation.

I was right. My respect for the distance kept me honest in my training. I cut no corners and took no shortcuts. On race day, I had butterflies in my stomach, but over the course of the many miles I had run in training, I had banished my fears. I felt ready.

And so I was. I ran a very good race, better than I expected. And most important, I enjoyed myself. I knew I would be back.

Can this approach work for you? Perhaps, though most runners decide to push themselves in shorter distances, and many decide against ever running the marathon. Indeed, I could have framed the question entirely differently. Instead of thinking that a 5K would not be worthwhile because I would not be a competitive runner, I could have challenged myself to run as fast as I could, regardless of whatever anyone else did. In fact, this is usually the only approach that really works, because it focuses on the only thing entirely in your own control. But I chose a different path.

My goal here is not to talk you into choosing any particular distance to race, whether it's your first or your 100th race. Instead, I ask that you think about the distance and whether it's right for you, emotionally and physically. Consider *why* you want to run it, *how* you would train for it, and *how* you would plan to run it. Your answers to these questions should lead you to the right race distance.

Standard Races

While race distances can and do vary greatly, the vast majority of races cover standard distances. Here is a list of the most common race distances, with my own opinion on the pros and cons of each.

5K. This is the standard race distance, and it is far and away the most popular race distance in the US. In 2022, there were more than 35,000 5K races in the US, with over 2.5 million total participants. There's a reason for this: a 5K is a race that almost anyone can finish. Equal to 3.1 miles, this distance can usually be walked in about an hour, although the world record for the race is currently an amazing 12 minutes, 35.36 seconds, or just over 4 minutes per mile.[24]

In all likelihood, your race would be somewhere between the fastest and the slowest, and you can challenge yourself as much or as little as you would like. If you plan to push yourself hard, however, be forewarned: many experienced runners consider the 5K to be perhaps the most challenging road race distance *minute for minute*. The race is too short to really settle into a pace, like in a marathon, and too long for a sprint, like in a 100-meter track race. So if you run the 5K fast, plan to suffer throughout.

10K. This is a more challenging race than the 5K, but also a distance that most participants can cover, especially if they are able to run at least part of it. The longer distance also provides a potentially more scenic route, as the extra miles allow race directors to connect more sites. While there are many 5Ks to choose from, however, you may not have quite as many convenient options for running a 10K near you.

Ten Miler. This, to me, is a great race because it strikes a balance between endurance and power. Fast runners can still cover the miles at a strong pace, while runners like me who have more endurance than speed can also find this race challenging.

Half-Marathon. I've always thought that this race was so oddly and unfortunately named. I can think of no other road race that is defined as being a portion of another race. It would

---

24 Set by the Ugandan runner Joshua Cheptegei in August 2020.

be like being referred to only as the brother or sister of your older sibling.

But this distance of 13.1 miles deserves its own star billing. It's a good test of endurance, giving finishers a great sense of accomplishment. But compared to its big sibling, it doesn't require as much preparation, does not take so much time to finish, and does not leave you as sore afterward. For many racers, this distance offers all the upsides of a longer race without the drawbacks. Because of that, it has become one of the most popular race distances in the US.

Marathon. I'm biased, as you may have guessed by now. I love the marathon. It forces you to give more than you think you can and rewards you by showing you how much you have to give. For my money, there is no race that can match the sense of satisfaction that finishing a marathon can provide.

The downsides, however—real or potential—are many. Overuse and repetitive stress injuries are common among marathoners, and preparing for the race takes a toll not just on the runner's body, but on their whole life, as social and family activities often take a back seat to a marathoner's training schedule. If you're going to run a marathon, it's a good idea to get buy-in first from your family and to pick a race that won't conflict with any other important events that are already scheduled.

Ultramarathon. There's a saying in running: any idiot can run a marathon, but it takes a special kind of idiot to run an ultra. Being that kind of idiot myself, I can attest to the truth of that.

An ultra is technically any distance that exceeds 26.2 miles, but most ultras fall into several specific distances: the 50K, the 50-miler, the 100K, and the 100-miler. Beyond that, there are 24-hour races and more. Basically, if you can conceive of a distance that no one would dare run, there's probably a race of that distance out there somewhere.

An ultra is for experienced racers who feel the need to challenge themselves to the very edge of what their bodies and minds can safely handle, and sometimes beyond. Race locales are often a great attraction; ultras are most often run on trails in beautiful parks and natural settings. Despite the risk of tripping, running on trails might also produce fewer injuries than running on roads because of the generally softer surfaces, the more varied way the body has to move over the terrain, and the slower pace that most ultra-runners settle into.

Strange as this may sound, running an ultra may not be as hard as you might think. Moving up from the 10K to the marathon requires the body to undergo significant transformations, most importantly from burning mostly stored carbohydrates to burning stored fat. Once the body has made these adaptations, moving from the marathon to an ultra requires only that it be done for longer periods. That's something the body can generally handle with less hard work than it took to get into marathon shape to begin with.

The downsides to running ultras are the possible damage to the heart that I mentioned earlier—something that has not been conclusively proven, but which may be of concern—and the way that the sport can easily dominate a person's life. Ultra-running tends to just not be a sport for many participants. It defines who they are, and it dominates their schedules.

For me, running ultras became too much. After running a half-dozen 50-milers and a 100K, I thought that the next logical step would be to run a 100-miler, but then something strange happened. I decided that I just didn't want to. Running a 100-miler requires running all through the night, pushing your body and mind to the point where hallucinations are common. This just didn't sound appealing to me. I know and respect runners who feel very differently, and maybe someday I'll change my mind, but I doubt it. As I told my friends, any mental health issues that I need to resolve could be handled in a marathon. After that, I should stop running and get a therapist.

Race Locations

Once you you've picked a distance, you need to pick a specific race. If you run with a group, that choice might be made for you already, since you could simply sign up for a race that your running friends are planning to do. I can think of no better way to enter the world of racing than in the company of your running pals. Training together, getting to the race start en masse, perhaps running the whole way together, and finally meeting up and celebrating together at the finish line will give you a sense of community that is difficult to fully explain to anyone who hasn't experienced it. It's why so many of us sign up for race after race, year after year.

There are more choices for you to make beyond what your local group has targeted, however. In fact, there is a world of races out there. You can look up races by country if you want an excuse to travel. But the more exotic the travel, the more carefully you might have to plan for it.

If you are traveling across time zones, and especially overseas, you need to consider how your travel and changes in altitude could affect your performance. If you head west, it may not be hard to get up early for a race if you don't try to adjust to the new time zone, but be aware that you might still have difficulty adjusting.

There is also the question of gear. My fear is that the airline will lose my bag and I'll be left without my shoes and clothes, so I make sure to bring my racing essentials as carry-on baggage.

Generally, I pick destination races to run for fun, and I use local races to aim for performance goals. After all, if I've traveled halfway around the world, I want to not just have fun in the race, but to also enjoy the country after crossing the finish line. If achieving a race goal would leave me too tired and sore to explore a new country and culture, I would consider that a lost opportunity. This is particularly true if I've got nonrunning family or friends with me who have cheered me on, but who would now like to go sightseeing. Of course, if your goal is to set a new personal record, you can target the fastest racecourses in the world, like the London and Berlin Marathons.

TRAINING FOR YOUR RACE

I don't intend this book to be a training guide for the event you've chosen—there are plenty of those guides out there. But we can take a moment now to briefly outline what a training plan should look like, and how to build one yourself, especially for longer races.

The first thing you should do after signing up for a race is circle the race date on a calendar, and then start counting backward from that date. The period right before your race is your time to rest up and get ready, referred to as the taper, when you wind down your training. This period lasts between one and three weeks, depending on the length of your target race. During those weeks, you will steadily decrease your training load. For a three-week marathon taper, for example, you would cut each week's training volume by 50 percent.

Next, to build your training plan, you would circle the date on your calendar right before the taper would begin. This would be the date of your last long training run —the longest run of your training cycle. You would then move backward on the calendar from weekend to weekend, filling in a long run on each that is slightly less than the one that follows, until your long run mileage countdown reaches your current long run distance.

The total number of weeks this process takes in your calendar is your training schedule. Now you have to fill in the weekdays in between your long runs with the rest of your program: shorter training runs, tempo runs, speed-work, cross-training, strength training, and whatever else you might want to include, like yoga.

And that's it, at least for a basic training plan. While much of training theory is based on science, as my mother would have said, it's not rocket science. You can use a coach, find a training plan online, run with a club, or write a plan yourself, but the idea is basically the same.

JEFF'S RULE OF TWO-THIRDS, PART I

All coaches agree that in preparing for a long distance race, you need to build up your running mileage. How much you need to build it up, however, is a matter of debate. In deciding how far your last long run before you race should be, you should consider both the race distance and your personal goals.

For races up to the half marathon, it's often recommended to do overage, that is, to exceed the race distance in training. So, for example, for a 10-mile race, you may want to end your hard training with a 12- or 14-mile run. By overpreparing, you will ensure that your body can handle the distance on race day. The only remaining question is how fast you can run it.

For the marathon, this approach runs into problems. If you aim to exceed the marathon's 26.2-mile distance in training, you will be putting a lot of stress on your body and potentially creating some damage. The question is whether any cardiovascular benefit that you may gain by running that far is outweighed by the risk of injury. For all except elite athletes—and often for them as well—the answer is to keep the runs shorter and avoid injuries.

Here's a good rule of thumb: whatever the race distance, if your goal is simply to finish the race, your last long run should be at least two-thirds of the race distance. So, 4 miles in preparation for the 10K (6.2 miles), 7 miles for the 10-miler, and 18 miles for the marathon. Less than that can leave you unprepared, while more than that might be more training than your goal requires.

If you are aiming to run fast, your last long run should be two miles over the race distance for races up to and including the half-marathon. For the marathon, I would recommend at least one

20-mile run in training—and several, if you have time—but no more than 23 miles.

My one real piece of advice on training for your race is this: take your race seriously and try to avoid cutting corners. For every workout you skip, you've raised the risk of not being able to finish your race or of getting injured just a little bit higher. You may get away with it for a while, but in my experience, it catches up with you eventually.

I understand that sometimes life gets in the way of our best intentions, and that we sometimes may need to take a calculated gamble on race day when we couldn't cross every "t" and dot every "i" in training. On those days, I adjust my race expectations and hope for the best.

If I am truly unable to prepare for a race, I may decide to skip that event. On those occasions, I think of my registration not as the purchase of a race slot, but as the purchase of an option. Most days I can exercise that option to race, but there are times, for whatever reason, when I may be unable to. On those unfortunate days, I consider my unused entry fee a contribution to the sport.

But otherwise, I aim to get to the start line as prepared as possible. That, to me, is the definition of taking the race seriously.

There is another reason to follow this advice that's less about performance and injury risk than it is about my personal philosophy. When you race, particularly when you participate in the longer races, you are among a group of people who have all trained hard for this event. Many of them have made sacrifices and have overcome serious obstacles. Some are obvious, as when you see racers with prosthetics or in wheelchairs. Some obstacles are less obvious, including emotional or mental health challenges, but are just as significant. Participating in this event, and completing it, will be a very meaningful event in their lives.

I believe that we honor the sport and all its participants when we prepare properly for our race and give it our best. In doing so, we uphold the best tradition of sport not only on that race day, but also on all race days that have come before.

I don't mean to say that there's no room for fun in racing—I love seeing people run in costume—but even then, I believe that they are doing something that they've planned and prepared for, and I can honor that as well. But to be cavalier about the race, to come to it unprepared, strikes me as diminishing the event for everyone.

This explains why runners hate cheaters. There are some runners who cut the course, or even jump in late, missing miles of the race, and then cross the finish line and go to collect their finisher's medal. When these people claim to have won the race, as has happened on occasion,[25] they are stealing the victory from another runner who should have won it. That is

---

[25] Most famously, there was Rosie Ruiz, who in 1980 was declared the winner of the Boston Marathon, only to have her title stripped when it was discovered that she had not run the whole course. Former House Speaker Paul Ryan claimed in 2012 to have run a sub-3-hour marathon when in fact he had run his only marathon in 4:01. That's more perplexing, since Ryan's actual race time was entirely respectable, and had he been honest, runners still would have appreciated the effort. But Ruiz and Ryan both wanted credit and respect for something they did not actually achieve.

clearly a wrongful act. But if they are far back in the pack, you might ask what harm it does to anyone else. The answer is that by getting a finisher's medal and claiming to have completed the race when they did not in fact do so, they have tarnished the accomplishment of everyone else who worked so hard to be able to earn the right to say that. To me, and for many others, that is wrong.

THE LIMITS OF SELFISHNESS

This might sound like an odd thing to say, but race day is the one time I believe that you are entitled to be unashamedly selfish. It's your moment to pursue your dream, one that you might have trained months for. I believe that you have a right to expect that, for this brief period, the world should revolve around you. From your dinner the night before, through race morning and until you cross the finish line, your needs should come first.

Within reasonable limits, of course. You also have obligations to those around you to make sure that this doesn't get out of control. Here are some guidelines to make sure that you don't step over the line:

Don't ask for more than you need. Try to minimize the burden that you put on everyone around you. Take care of as many of the logistics of racing as you can, and ask for as little help from those around you as possible. Putting your own needs first for race day does not mean you can be a prima donna.

Return the favor. I don't recommend treating your relationships transactionally, but it might help to imagine that you are living with a point system. You earn points by being supportive of those around you and spend your points when you ask for their understanding and support on race day. It's always a good idea to try to earn more points than you use by supporting others as much, or more, than they need to support you. If you are in a relationship with another racer, then this means supporting them on their race weekend as much or more than you need to be supported on yours.

Don't go to the well too often. Although I focus on myself on race day, I know that there are probably only a limited number of times that I could expect people to agree to this. I prioritize my races, and I make clear that there's no need for them to come out to support me in what I consider my less-important races. I figure that if they know that I don't expect them to get up early and come cheer for me for every race I enter, then they won't be resentful when I sign up for yet another event.

PREPARING FOR RACE DAY

You've successfully made your way through your training plan, and now, as you begin your taper, it is time for you to give some serious thought to your expectations on race day. If your aim is to simply finish the race, then pace is of little concern to you as long as you beat the time limit. If this is your first race at a particular distance, then you are in a unique position: as long as you finish the race, you will be guaranteed a personal record, or a "PR" in racers' lingo. That's something that you will never again be sure of getting in that race. If you are hoping to challenge yourself with a time goal, however, you need to consider several factors.

First, consider your past performances. If you've raced at that same distance before, you may have a sense of what to expect in your upcoming race. If you're about to participate in a new race distance but have raced other distances before, you may consider consulting a pace predictor chart. These graphs have a horizontal axis of common race distances, and vertical axis of finishing times. The graphs are based on the principle that we all run faster at shorter distances than longer distances, and that our speed diminishes at a steady and predicable rate as we run longer and longer. Using this principle, the chart predicts finishing times across a range of races.[26]

To estimate what you may expect to run in your first marathon after having raced a 10K earlier in the year, all you would need to do is look up your 10K finishing time on the chart, and then trace your finger to the right until you are in the marathon column, and there is the marathon finishing time that you may expect, based on your 10K time.

A pace predictor chart is a useful tool, but it should not be taken as gospel truth. It is based on several assumptions, including a consistent and successful training cycle from one race to the next. It also does not take genetic predisposition

---

[26] A standard pace predictor chart can be found here: https://www. runningfoundation.com/Pace_Charts/RaceTimePredictorChart.html. htm.

into account, such as my tendency to run relatively stronger in longer races than shorter races.[27]

Interestingly, a pace predictor chart can also help you identify areas to focus on in training. If your marathon times suggest that you should be running a faster 5K than you have been, you should work more on speed. Conversely, if your 5K pace predicts a faster marathon, then you should do more endurance training, because you have speed, but you are just not able to hold it long enough.

Second, look back on your training pace for various workouts, especially the most recent ones. There's a phrase in coaching that applies here: train the way you'll race, and race the way you've trained. In other words, work hard enough in training to simulate a pace or effort level that you'll expect to be able to hold on race day, and then on race day, try to run near the pace that you were able to maintain in training.

This sounds sensible enough, but you'd be surprised at how many people I've met who bolted out from the start line on race day at a pace that I *knew* for a fact they'd never achieved in training. I could only look at their race day pace as a kind of magical thinking; that somehow they would become a different person

---

27 This, in turn, is based on differences in our muscle fiber types. Not all muscle fibers are exactly the same; scientists have identified fibers that are referred to as quick twitch and slow twitch fibers. The former are more responsible for explosive movements, while the latter support longer aerobic efforts. We all have both types, but often in different amounts, as determined by our genes. Your abilities as a sprinter or marathoner are determined in part by how much of each type of fiber you are born with. Of course, your training will play a big role in this as well.

on race day than they'd been in training. Invariably, the race soon proved otherwise.

I should add a caveat here: while your training pace should be a good predictor of what you could accomplish in your race, you can expect to be probably at least a little bit faster on race day than you were in training. That's due to several factors.

If you trained and tapered correctly, your fitness should be peaking on race day, leaving you primed for your best run. On race day, you will probably also be more rested than you were at any point during training, as you've been tapering for a week or more beforehand.

Further, you will get more logistical support on race day than you probably ever had in training, in the form of aid stations stocked with water, sports drink, and perhaps snacks as well.

You will also benefit from the excitement that comes from being part of a field of racers, where the energy is almost palpable and you take in the cheering from spectators, who probably don't know how much their encouragement really helps us.

LOOKING DOWN THE HOME STRETCH

With your training complete, your taper almost finished, and your race goal in mind, you are now ready to begin the final phase of your preparation: the last few days before the race.

If you follow a good pre-race plan, you will put yourself in a position to do your best on race day. But don't panic if you aren't able to nail all of this perfectly; some of my best races came after I had a less-than-perfect final preparation. Still, let's aim to put the odds in our favor by making this as picture-perfect as possible.

Prioritize your sleep. First, aim to get a good night's sleep two nights before the race. So, if your race is on Sunday, try your best to get as much quality sleep as possible on Friday night. Go to bed early and try to arrange things so that you can sleep in as late as possible. By getting a good night's sleep, then, you will have created a "sleep reserve," so even if you don't sleep well on the night before a race because of nerves or for any other reason, you will still be fine on race day.

I'm recalling now the night before one of my marathons. Everything had gone right, and I settled down to bed in the early evening. I drifted off to sleep congratulating myself on my discipline in following my plan. I woke up on race day feeling refreshed and ready, but when I looked at the clock, I saw that it was just 1:30 a.m.! I had slept for only a couple of hours, and now I was too excited to go back to sleep. Still, I didn't panic because I had a good night's sleep the night before, so I knew I'd be fine later. And I was.

Limit your activities. Plan not just your sleep, but also your activities on those final few days. If possible, pick up your race number two days before. That way you can enjoy the big race expo, if there is one, and avoid big crowds and long lines that may come later. If you are unable to get your number earlier and can only get it the day before the race, try not to spend too much time doing that. If there's a big expo and you really want to see it, which is one of the most fun things about participating in a big race, put a time limit on being there. You may not realize it, but spending a lot of time wandering a race expo can fatigue your legs and leave you tired on race day.

If you are in a different city or even country, try to avoid sightseeing the day before the race, as this could also fatigue your legs. Leave that for after the race. A great option might be to go see a movie instead or even do some easy laps in a pool.

Eat early. Eat your pre-race dinner early so that you give yourself plenty of time to digest. With any luck, you will be able to eliminate before you have to leave for the race the next day. Don't overdo it. Carb loading is often misunderstood; technically, this requires carb depletion before loading, which means exercising to failure, and then pushing food into the vacuum created by your fuel-burn. Since you shouldn't exercise to failure right before a race, you won't need to carb load. Just eat a comfortable amount of food. If you get hungry again later, you could have an energy bar or other light snack.

Upon waking on race morning, I eat my breakfast as soon as possible in order to give myself plenty of time to digest before the race begins. I make sure to eat only simple foods that I've tested already before other races and long runs, and I avoid overeating. As a rule of thumb, I aim to have less than 500 calories. Some oatmeal or a bagel, a banana, and some juice are more than enough.

Prepare the night before. Before you go to bed, lay out everything you need on race day so that you don't have to try to find anything in the morning as you're rushing to get out the door. I put pins on my race number and leave it next to my shirt, and I lay all my clothes on the floor by my bed next to my racing shoes. I put anything else I need on the side table: sports gels, gloves, hat, sunglasses, and any other clothes. I leave nothing to chance.

Since most races are in the fall or spring, weather can be unpredictable. I save old sweatshirts and track pants to use as throwaways, and I wear a large garbage bag with a hole poked in the top as a poncho. This keeps me dry before the race if it's wet out and helps hold in my body heat if it's cold. I wear it right up until I hear the starting gun, when, Superman-like, I tear it away and fly off.

I also wear my extra clothes as long as possible before packing them in a bag provided by the race for gear-check.

On getting to the race start, I head right to the port-a-john line, knowing that even if I don't need to use it yet, I probably will need to by the time I get to the front of the line.

WARMING UP FOR YOUR RACE

As a rule of thumb, the shorter the race, the longer your warm-up should be. That's because the shorter the race, the faster the pace should be right off the start line, so you need to be ready. For a 5K, for example, I'll do some easy running, then some drills, then some short striders, which are like sprints, and finally, some stretching. This process may take almost as much time as it will take me to run the whole race.

In contrast, I do hardly any warm-up for the marathon. I may do some easy squats, lunges, and twists to warm up my legs and back, but I won't spend more than a few minutes on this. My strategy is to just start the race running at a controlled pace, and then ease into a faster pace as my body warms up. Knowing that I'll be out there for several hours makes a more extensive warm-up unnecessary.

Then it's time to head to the start line. I've known racers who try to get as close to the front as possible, but unless you're a fast runner, I consider this a bad idea, both for others and for you. If you are not fast enough to be in the lead pack, you'll just get in their way once the race begins. And if you can't keep up, it's no fun getting passed by runners—maybe hundreds or even thousands of them.

It's much better instead to be among runners who plan to run a pace similar to your own. For races that assign runners to corrals based on their predicted finishing times, that's easy to figure out. For all other races, it's best to plant yourself somewhere in the middle. If you're among runners who are slower than you are, you'll have the joy of passing others as you move up in the crowd. Eventually, all runners, like water, find their level.

SETTING YOUR RACE GOAL

Let's do this thought experiment: What would a successful race look like to you? Are you aiming to just finish, or do you have a time goal?

I consider this a trick question, because the answer is instead of having just one goal for your race, you should keep several in mind. This view is based on the Hierarchy of Needs established by the psychologist Abraham Maslow, in which Maslow identified five ascending motivating factors for humans.[28] His pyramid of needs moves from physiological needs at the bottom, to safety, love/belonging, esteem, and finally, at the pinnacle, self-actualization.

---

28 Abraham H. Maslow, "A Theory of Human Motivation," *Psychological Review* 50, no. 4 (1943): 370–96.

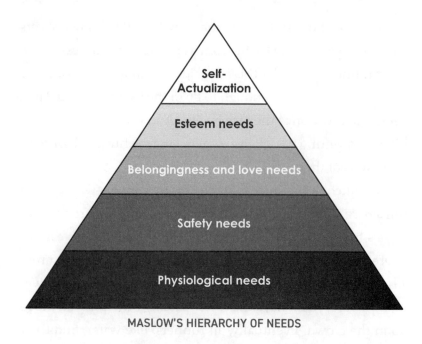

MASLOW'S HIERARCHY OF NEEDS

My Racer's Hierarchy of Needs would look like this, in ascending order, starting from the bottom:

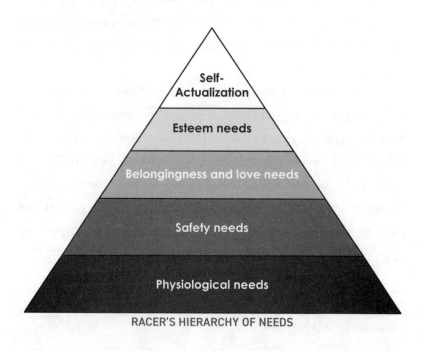

RACER'S HIERARCHY OF NEEDS

THINK LIKE A **RUNNER**

When I race, I head out with a realistic finishing time in mind, based on my recent training experience. My goal is rarely a specific number; instead, it is usually a range, based on my best and worst training days leading up to the race. Only rarely has my final time been much different from what I would have expected.

This goal is not carved in stone, however. Once the starter's gun goes off, I let the race unfold and I periodically ask my body how it's feeling. The answers will determine which of these goals are realistic. I always aim to meet the entry-level goal of not getting hurt; after that, anything is possible.

RUNNING YOUR RACE

For me, there is hardly any other moment that could compare with the few minutes before a race. I'm packed in with thousands, sometimes tens of thousands, of other people, all eagerly awaiting the horn or starter's gun that will send us on our way. The energy is fantastic. Everyone jokes, laughs, sings the national anthem, and cheers as they await the start.

And then we're off! Except we're not. There's usually a false surge, which grinds to a stop as the crowd in front of us slowly makes its way over the electronic starting mat. Expect this, and don't get frustrated. Soon our race will begin in earnest. Acknowledge the cheers and smiles from the friends and families lining the roadway—they should know that they're appreciated.

It's common for runners to grumble about how jammed up they are at the beginning of a race and how long it took until the crowd opened up and they were able to speed up into their planned pace. Over the years, I've come to see a bright side to this. It's very easy and tempting to start a race too quickly. In smaller races, where I can run as fast as I'd like from the very beginning, I have to focus on not running faster than I should. In a big race, however, the crowd forces me to run conservatively in the beginning, which can set me up for success later on.

BEGINNING RACE STRATEGIES

Knowing the course helps with anticipation and strategy. I've got a friend who actually counts all the turns in a racecourse so that he'll know how many of these he will have to negotiate on race day. I actually don't mind being a bit surprised on the racecourse—for me, this discovery is part of what makes racing fun—but I do want to know beforehand if there are any significant hills on the course, and where they might be, so that I can pace myself accordingly. I'm especially leery of any hills that have earned their own nicknames, like Heartbreak Hill in the Boston Marathon, or Hurricane Point in the Big Sur Marathon. U-turns on the course can also disrupt my pace, and I like to know how many of those I can expect.

Racers often talk about their splits, which are their times for each of the miles or kilometers in a race. So, for example, if your goal was to finish a marathon in less than three hours, you would need to average split times of 6 minutes, 51 seconds per mile. The Holy Grail of running is to run a slight negative split. That is, to run the second half of the race a bit faster than the first. This indicates that you've run a smart, controlled race. If you ran the second half slower than the first, you probably slowed down from fatigue, which shows that you either did not train as hard in preparing for the race as you should have, or that you started out faster than you should have and simply ran out of gas.

Running near-even splits is the goal, but some courses do not lend themselves to running even splits because they have at least several hills. In this case, your split times may be all over the map, as you run slower on the uphills and faster on the downhills. On such courses, instead of trying to run even splits, your goal should be to run at an even effort level. Your downhills will naturally be faster than your uphills, but it will all average out to a good overall pace in the end.

As I make my way over a racecourse, I try to plan out as many things as I can in order to leave as little to chance as possible. I call this "micro-strategizing." For example, when I come to an aid station in a big race, my strategy is to pass the earlier tables and head to the end of the line. This will let me avoid the crush of runners who swarm around the first few volunteers. When I near the far table, I try to make eye contact with a specific volunteer, and sometimes I'll even point to them, all to let them know that I'm coming to them to grab a cup. This tends to make the handoff smoother.

At this point, some runners will squeeze the cup to form a funnel that they can use to pour the water or sports drink into their mouth as they run. I choose to walk instead as I drink. This only takes a few seconds—I'm still moving forward, after all—and it makes it much easier to for me to drink the whole cup. After getting fully refreshed, I can easily make up the few seconds I've lost.

JEFF'S RULE OF TWO-THIRDS, PART II

Learning how to pace yourself properly during a race is one of the hardest things to achieve in running. I've met elite runners—people who were vying for a spot on the American Olympic marathon team—who told me that they only rarely got it right. "I felt good at the start," one told me, "I thought, 'maybe this is my day,' and so I went out too fast. I paid for that later in the race."

I've been there myself. You think, sure, this is faster than I've ever run in training, but maybe I'm just feeling really good, and this is what I'm really capable of doing. It's a form of magical thinking. Or, to use the words of the late Federal Reserve Bank chairman Alan Greenspan, it's a case of "irrational exuberance."

While there's no set rule on how fast you should run in a race, I've found a simple formula to help ensure that you don't ruin your race and go out too fast. Run the first two thirds of your race conservatively, at a pace no faster than a little bit slower that your fastest pace in training. Fast, but not overly ambitious.

Then, on reaching the two-thirds mark of the race, do a quick assessment of how you're feeling. If you still feel great, go for it! Speed up. If you misjudged your energy reserve and start to peter out, you're still close enough to the finish line to complete the race, even if you have to slow down a bit. If, however, you are indeed having a great day, you will not have run so slow that you'll regret not running harder earlier, and you still have enough mileage left to end up with a great finishing time.

I sum up this approach with the phrase, "Put 'em in the bank, then check the tank." That simply means cover a significant part of the race and then assess how you feel.

This guideline seems to hold true for races of all distances. So, that moment of truth would roughly be at the 2-mile mark in a 5K, the 4-mile mark in a 10K, and the 18-mile mark in the marathon.

Whatever your race strategy, at least be aware of what you're doing and be *purposeful*. If you decide to take a chance by going out fast, do so with the awareness that if you misjudged what your body can do, you might have to drop out of the race. Sometimes the possibility of setting a new personal record is worth the risk of not completing the race—as long as you consciously make that choice.

THE WALL

In almost every race, there's a point at which you would rather not be running anymore. The early excitement has burned off, and now the race just seems hard. This is especially true of the long races.

You're probably familiar with the Wall, that dreaded point in the marathon, usually somewhere around miles 18 to 21, where it feels like the wheels might be coming off. This can be the result of a physiological crisis, where the body's reserves of carbohydrates have been used up and the body has not learned to burn its high-energy fat stores.

In essence, hitting the Wall indicates a flaw in a runner's training or racing plan. If you have not done enough long runs in training, the body is not prepared to burn fat in the race, and you will have run out of available stored carbohydrates after about two and a half hours. Or, if you start out your race too fast, the body will burn through its carbohydrate stores too quickly, leaving you equally depleted of fuel at about the same place. Either way, hitting the Wall is not an inevitable part of racing; smart training and disciplined racing should help you avoid it.

But the Wall can be more than a physiological event; it can be an emotional pit. Road racing can be very mentally taxing, and the longer the race, the more of an emotional challenge it can be. By the time most runners hit miles 18 to 21 in a race, they've been out there working hard for two or three hours, and they've still got another hour or more to go. Their bodies are complaining, and they find it harder and harder to focus on the task at hand. This can be the low point of the race.

Working through the Wall

There are strategies that we can employ at this point to help us through. As I mentioned elsewhere, I tend to think in analogies, and here's one that works for me: skating. I think of running the first half of the marathon as if I were skating on a big frozen lake. I glide almost effortlessly over the smooth, even ice. But then, somewhere around that 18- to 21-mile mark, the ice thins over the shoreline, and I hit gravel. I don't panic, though, because I know that if I can get past this rough patch, there's smooth ice up ahead. Then, almost invariably, I do make it back onto that smooth ice, and I am able glide to the finish line.

I encourage you to use this image, or think of another one that could work for you when you're experiencing the Wall. Or create a mantra, or pick just a single word, that will empower you when you repeat it.

TALKING TO MYSELF

Having a good mantra is like having your own cheerleader.

Many people have heard of mantras, but few know their origin. Mantra is a Sanskrit term meaning "a tool for thinking." While they were traditionally used to focus the mind to achieve religious and spiritual development during meditation, they can help us focus during racing.

Sports psychologists say that mantras in general should be short, positive statements that help instruct and motivate you to give your best. They could be as simple as a reminder to "Run strong," "Attack the hill," "Breathe easy," or "Hold your pace." Olympic medalist and marathon champion Deena Kastor repeated "Define yourself" as she raced, and ultramarathon legend Scott Jurek reminded himself, "This is what you came for."

I have several mantras that I rely on. "Forward motion" reminds me that as long as I keep moving toward the finish line, I'll eventually get there. "You've worked for this" reminds me of all the effort I've put into training, that I'm prepared for this, and that I don't want all that hard work to go to waste.

Some mantras I take from the world around me. I call them "found mantras." Traffic signs are a surprisingly good source of motivation. I take "Yield" and "Stop" signs as personal challenges, and I find myself silently answering, "I will *not!*" When I see a 25-mile-per-hour speed limit sign, I try to live up to the sign's optimism by speeding up.

Other mantras are less about motivation and more about general life lessons. A small metal tag I once saw lying in the street had the inscription "Record and Detach," and though it just referred to a model number, I took it to mean that I should be aware but stay calm if I encountered any setbacks or problems.

My favorite found mantra, though, is one that I saw flashing on a large electronic road sign. "Expect Delays," it warned, and I thought, yes, that pretty much sums up life.

You may anticipate needing different mantras for different parts of the race as your emotional needs change. Imagine how you'll feel at each part, perhaps based on how you've felt during your long runs, and find what works for you.

Another strategy is to bargain with yourself to keep going. Runners often promise themselves a big, delicious, decadent meal after the race. Cheeseburgers with a side order of fries and a large milkshake often seem to do the trick. But bribes don't have to be limited to food; you can promise yourself a massage, jewelry, a trip, a phone upgrade, or anything that you could imagine, if only you'll keep moving.

Sometimes the payoff has to be more immediate. I've promised myself walk breaks and fuel breaks to keep running. I've broken down my running to taking ten steps at a time, and I just keep repeating the process. In more extreme moments, I've even told myself that I'd consider dropping out after reaching the next mile marker. Of course, at that mile marker, I usually decide to keep going to the next one, and so on, using that same promise again and again.

Some people try to use the people around them to keep going. A friend of mine throws an imaginary lasso around the runner in front of him and lets himself get pulled along. Similarly, I'll pick one person to latch on to, and just try to keep up with them.

Striking up a conversation with the runner next to you can also help. In all likelihood, they're struggling as much as you are. By giving and getting encouragement, you both will end up finding a reserve of energy that will get you through to the end.

You can keep all of these strategies in your mental toolbox and deploy each of them as needed. Sometimes, one may work where another one doesn't, even if the other strategy has worked well before.

PACE GROUPS

Many big races use pacers to help runners stay on track to achieve their goals. Pacers run a very precise race to achieve a specific pre-announced finishing time, and anyone who wants to finish in that same time could just stay close to that pacer and not worry about checking their watches. They could also enjoy the energy that comes from running with a group.

Running with a pace group in a race is free. You don't need to sign up, and you are not committed to staying with a group. You can spot them at the starting line; they'll be holding a light stick with a balloon or banner attached to the top on which is written their goal finishing time.

Pacers tend to be very reliable. They commit to finishing within a minute of their target time, and to run as close to even splits along the way as possible. It's a little like throwing a dart across the city and hitting the bull's eye. And yet they do it.

To make the best use of pacers, I recommend this approach:

Don't count on the pacer to make an unrealistic dream come true. A pacer cannot help you run a faster race than you have trained for. If your plan is to rely on the pacer to help you achieve an unrealistic goal, you'll be sorely disappointed.

If you lose touch with a pace group, don't try to catch up all at once. At some point during the race, you may need a potty break, or you might linger at an aid station. If you lose contact with the pace group, do not sprint to catch up with them. This could wear you out unnecessarily. Instead, speed up just a little and reel them in slowly over the next mile or so.

Think of pacers as moving landmarks. Pacers are like moving clocks. If you want to finish a marathon in less than four hours, you know you're on pace if the four-hour pace group doesn't pass you. You could also plant yourself between pace groups to achieve a time between the two.

You can use different pacers. You have no loyalty to the group, so you can shift up or down between pace groups as necessary. If you start with the one group and you feel great, perhaps you can catch up to the next one. Or, if things aren't going so well, you can drop back to the next group behind you.

A quick note on etiquette: pacers love to race, and they usually love talking with runners, but the groups can get big and crowded. Chat with your pacers, but give them a little elbow room. They'll appreciate it.

Knowing When Enough Is Enough

There are times when all the bribes and promises in the world won't work, and this just isn't your day. Perhaps an injury hasn't healed, or you just feel too tired and sore to go on. At those moments, dropping out of the race might be the best—and smartest—thing to do.

In 1982, Julie Moss was competing in a relatively new event, the Kona Ironman Triathlon. The Ironman distance combined a 2¼-mile swim, a 112-mile bike ride, and a 26.2-mile marathon-distance run into a single grueling event. Moss, 23, was winning the race, and was literally just a dozen or so feet from sealing her victory. Except that she was completely exhausted and fell to the ground. She pulled herself back up but fell again. And again. Another woman passed her, depriving her of victory, but still Moss struggled on. Unable to stand, she crawled across the finish line. Medics then rushed to her side, now able to render help without getting her disqualified.

The event was broadcast on network TV, and viewers around the world watched her struggle. Moss's achievement became legendary and inspired athletes for decades to come. She is a hero.

And yet....

As much as I am inspired by Moss's story (even now, as I write about it, I can feel goosebumps), I wonder if the medical crew did the right thing by not jumping in as soon as she fell. Yes, it would have been heartbreaking to see her fail to win or even drop out of the race after getting within a hair's length of the finish line. But it would have been tragic if she had died trying to do so. [29]

With that in mind, we return to our first and perhaps most important rule: *Be smarter than you are brave.* I know that you have the determination and willpower to push yourself on when your body is telling you to stop, but you need to recognize that there are times when you need to be coldly clinical in

---

[29] Dying while running a marathon is a very rare event, but it does happen. From 2000 to 2009 there were over 3.7 million marathon participants in the United States. Of these, 28 people died. That's 0.00075 percent of the participating runners. Of these, 93 percent died of a heart attack or heart disease. Simon C. Mathews et al., "Mortality among Marathon Runners in the United States, 2000–2009," *American Journal of Sports Medicine* 40, no. 7 (July 2012): 1495–500.

viewing your situation, and sometimes the right thing to do is to quit the race.

I'm reminded of a scene from the old classic David Lean movie, *The Bridge on the River Kwai*. The character played by William Holden is an American prisoner of war in a Japanese work camp, and in one scene he's talking with a British prisoner about the captured British commander, played by Alec Guinness. The Brit tells Holden how brave Guinness is, but Holden is not comforted. "That's the kind of guts that can get us all killed,"[30] he says. By the end of the movie, his words prove prophetic.

Holden would have been a good marathoner. Be courageous when racing. Be heroic. Run through moderate pain—tendinitis, after all, never killed anyone. Run past fatigue and doubt. But don't ignore your body's warnings if it tells you that something is seriously wrong.

Elite runners know this rule. They drop out of races all the time because they know that finishing one race is not more important than keeping their body injury-free. For them, this is a crucial decision to make because their bodies are their livelihood. There is always another race. They know that stopping for the right reason is not a sign of weakness; it's a sign of discipline and intelligence. People who don't understand this are not true runners.

Here are some easy examples of severe warning signs that should send you to the medical tent:

- If you are feeling a very sharp, pinpoint pain in your foot, you may have a stress fracture. Continued running

---

30 David Lean, dir. *The Bridge on the River Kwai*, 1957, Horizon Pictures, distributed by Columbia Pictures.

can make that injury much, much worse, and can even risk permanent disfigurement.

- If you are dizzy and nauseous, you may be on the road to heat stroke or hyponatremia.
- If you experience tightness in the chest and pain down the left arm, you may be experiencing a heart attack.

If you get *any* of these symptoms, you should seek medical attention on the course at one of the aid stations.

In fact, if you have any doubt about what you should do, seek medical attention. You might only be experiencing a small problem, and you may be able to get back into the race after receiving a little bit of help and advice. But let an expert make that call.

PARTNER WITH YOUR BODY

Years ago, I was running in a local 10-mile race on a closed section of the George Washington Parkway. It's a beautiful tree-lined course that follows the Potomac River from Washington's estate at Mount Vernon north to the historic Old Town in Alexandria, Virginia. The route is almost entirely straight and mostly flat, making it a very fast course. My goal was to run just a few fast miles and then ease off for a comfortable finish. I meant it only to be a good workout in support of other race goals.

The race began, and I flew through the first mile. The second felt just as good, as did the third. I'd now basically met my goal for the race, but I was feeling strong, so I kept my fast pace through the fourth mile, and then the fifth.

I now found myself in a quandary. I had exceeded my goal for the day and could have slowed down, but I was also halfway to having a really good finishing time. If I was able to hold my pace, I might even be able to set a new personal record.

In the world of running, these moments don't come around that often. I should have been thrilled. But a small part of me was unhappy. I knew that by deciding to race hard the rest of the way, I was committing to a lot of discomfort. But I felt that I had no choice, really. I knew that if I threw away this opportunity, I would regret it later.

There's a saying in running that you often see printed on spectators' signs along the racecourse: pain is temporary, but pride is forever. So, I really never doubted what I would do. I kept running fast.

The last few miles were as difficult as I'd anticipated. My legs ached and my lungs burned, but I held my pace, and yes, I did set a new personal record. Later, when my breathing settled down and my legs began to recover, I was left only with the pride of my accomplishment.

BE OPPORTUNISTIC, PART II

The mindset of being opportunistic when you race synthesizes all of the strategies and rules of racing we've discussed already and returns us to a concept we reviewed earlier in Chapter Two. Train diligently, have an appropriate race plan, but listen to your body. Sometimes it might tell you that you need to slow down, or even stop racing. But sometimes, *sometimes*, it might tell you to push harder, that it is ready and willing to give a bit more than you were expecting. If you have one of those rare moments, as I did on that 10-mile course, don't waste it. Take advantage of the opportunity that's presented to you.

The flip side of being opportunistic, however, is to be willful. It took me years to realize that this is not a good trait. I believed firmly in being able to push my body harder and took to heart all the pithy phrases that are supposed to motivate us to excel, like "No pain, no gain," "Mind over matter," and "Pain is just weakness leaving the body." After all, none of us would ever finish a marathon if we stopped every time our bodies told us they felt uncomfortable. Stubbornness is an essential element of racing success.

The problem with this approach is that it assumes that you must be in opposition to your body, that you must make it bend to your will. In fact, your body is not your enemy. It is perfectly happy to help you cross a race finish line.

Instead of thinking of your body as being your enemy, you should look on your body instead as being your partner. An *active* partner. It will tell you when it feels ready to go harder, and also when it needs more rest. Listen to it, give it what it needs—proper training, good fuel, and enough rest—and in return it will give you everything that it can.

AFTER YOU FINISH

CROSSING THE FINISH LINE

For my money, there is nothing in life that compares to crossing a finish line, especially if you have given it all that you had. The sense of satisfaction and accomplishment is like nothing else that I've experienced.

Enjoy this feeling. You've earned it. But although the running is over, you've got other things to do now.

First, keep moving. You may feel like flopping down on the ground, but that's exactly what you should avoid. Right now—especially if you've run the longer distances—your legs are filled with waste products that are sitting there like garbage in a trash can waiting to be taken out. You want that cleared out, and walking will create a pumping action in your muscles that will accomplish just that.[31]

Second, thank as many volunteers as you can. No race could exist without their support, and some of them have been out there for many hours working to make our experience better, and they'll be out there after we've gone home. I'm very grateful to all of them, and I want them to know. I extend thanks as well to the police who monitor the intersections and try to ensure our safety. I've never regretted saying thanks.

Third, eat and drink, even if you don't feel like it. There's a 30-minute window immediately after you stop running when your body will jump-start the recovery process if you feed it a mix of carbohydrates (to replenish lost fuel) and proteins (to repair muscle). In addition, you are probably dehydrated, even if you were drinking on the course, especially if it was a hot day. So drink up as well.[32]

You may find that you are not only able to eat after a long race, but that you're actually ravenous. That could be a very

---

31 This is one reason why some big races put the gear retrieval and family reunion areas so far from the finish line. You may grumble about having to walk after running so hard, but it's for your own good.

32 To get an idea of how dehydrated you are after racing, weigh yourself before and after your race. Any weight loss will be due mostly to lost water that needs to be replaced. You should also take note of the color and odor of your urine. The more yellow and concentrated it is, the more likely you are to be dehydrated.

good sign, as it means that your brain did not see your race as a crisis that required it to shut down your gastrointestinal system. In other words, you did not run harder than your autonomous brain considered reasonable.

ASSESSING YOUR RACE EXPERIENCE

At this point, you'll probably begin the process of rating your experience. After all, you'll have to say something when your friends, family, and coworkers asked how the race went.

This question actually has two parts: how was the *race*, and how did *you* do? Often, there's one answer to both, but sometimes the answers are very different. I've had bad races on great courses. I've also had the reverse—where the aid stations were not set up by the time the runners got to them, or there was a lack of signage so we almost got lost, but I performed above my expectations.

In assessing my race performance, my respect for racing, and for the marathon in particular, has led me to this mindset: while I might have time goals for the race, every marathon is so challenging that simply finishing the race is a huge accomplishment. And any time I finish a marathon, even if I don't achieve my time goal, I should be happy with my effort. If I cannot be happy with a finish, then I should not race anymore.

Over the years, I've been challenged to live up to this way of thinking, and in doing so, I've had to modify it: all I can ask of myself on race day is, under all the circumstances—including my training, my injuries, the weather, the course, and whatever else may affect my race—did I give it my very best effort? If the answer is yes, then there is nothing else I could have asked of myself, and the race was a success.

This is true even of the races that I did not finish (DNF). And yes, there have been some of those. In fact, I'm prouder of some of those DNFs, in a way, than I am of my finishes. They are proof that I know my limits, and I had the discipline and intelligence to stop. I console myself with the knowledge that there will be another day. As the saying goes: Sometimes you're the windshield; sometimes you're the bug. In life, we have to learn to accept it all.

RECOVERY BEGINS

Soak in the post-race atmosphere. It's a heady mix of relief and joy, although sometimes tempered by disappointment. Enjoy the moment. There's not an endless supply of them, so each one is special.

You might be tempted to sit down and rest, but don't. Walking around will keep the blood moving through your legs, which will help with recovery.

Finally, after the post-race bagels and bananas have been eaten and washed down with water or sports drink (or, sometimes, chocolate milk![33]), it's time to go home. After getting clean, you can take a 10-minute ice bath to reduce inflammation in your legs, if you can stand it, or at least lie down with your legs elevated for a time to help blood drain out of your limbs.

---

33 In a happy occurrence that some might say is proof of God's love for us, scientists have discovered that chocolate milk is actually a perfect post-race replenishment drink after an endurance workout, as it is made up of a perfect balance of 3 to 4 grams of carbohydrate for every gram of protein. Kate Patton, "Should You Drink Chocolate Milk after a Workout?" *Cleveland Clinic Health Essentials*, December 20, 2020.

You may opt to get a post-race massage immediately after the race or a few days later. This is a great idea, but make sure that the therapist doesn't dig too deep. Your exertions have created microscopic tears in your muscle fibers, and you need time to heal. A vigorous deep-tissue massage will just make this worse. Instead, you should get a light massage, with the goal of flushing waste products out of the muscle tissue and enhancing circulation and restoring range of motion.

ANALYZING YOUR PERFORMANCE

If running a race was a bucket list adventure for you, then you should be proud of achieving your dream. Now you can return to your regular running life.

If you plan to continue racing, though, you should ask yourself if you're interested in improving. That's not a rhetorical question. Some people just enjoy the race experience and don't care at all about performance. A friend of mine calls such runners "race participants" rather than "racers." There's nothing wrong with that. In fact, you can switch between being one or the other, like a boxer taking on an easy opponent after fighting a tough one.

Perhaps you are a racer, but you've decided that challenging yourself on race day is enough. Your finishing time is less important than just trying your best. You are happy with how training fits into your life, and competing at this level on race day totally satisfies you. You see no need to change your routine, so you can probably skip the race analysis. I completely understand and respect that.

But if you are curious about whether you can get faster—and how much faster—now is the time to look back on your race experience and take what lessons you can from it. By analyzing your race, you will be able to figure out what worked and what did not and make necessary adjustments going forward.

Start by asking yourself if you hit the goals that you set beforehand. If so, then you may now consider setting a slightly more ambitious goal for your next race. Consider adjusting your training volume and intensity to see if you can lay the foundation for improvement, and then consider what a realistic but challenging new time goal could be.

But if you fell short of your goals on race day, let's try to figure out why. We'll begin by looking at your race preparation.

Race Preparation. Did you make it to the starting line as well prepared as you had hoped? Racing well depends in large part on how well you were able to mimic the race environment in training. If your training plan stressed your body in a carefully calibrated way, your body should have been prepared for the similar stress of race day. If you trained on hills, for example, you should have been ready for a hilly racecourse. If you were training for a marathon, your long runs should have prepared you mentally and physically for the challenge ahead.

Did your race plan adequately prepare you for the race that you ran? Think on where you had the most trouble in the race. Did you fizzle out on the hills, fail to hit your target speed, or run out of gas toward the end? Your answers will tell you whether your next training plan should include more hill-work, speed-work, or endurance-work.

Training. But perhaps the problem was not with your plan but with your ability to follow it. Did you miss any workouts because of work, family, or social commitments? If you didn't have enough time to fit in all the training you needed, perhaps you need a longer training cycle. Or, if your days seem too busy to get in all your training, perhaps you need to get creative with scheduling to make it all work. Run commuting, for example, may take longer than driving or taking public transportation, but if you can work out the details, you may find that this can end up being a time saver overall.

Or perhaps you just found it hard to get out the door to run. Answer this honestly, but don't let guilt or shame be a part of this. This process is not about blaming yourself; it's about getting answers and moving forward. If motivation was an issue and you trained alone, maybe running with a group would help. We all feel more committed to getting out for a run if we know that there are people waiting for us. If you were just bored, try new routes, or consider listening to music or a good podcast.

Remember, too, that the goal here is not to reach perfection; it's about just making improvements. Even a less-than-perfect training cycle can yield great results, and deviating from your training plan doesn't necessarily doom you to failure. If we were able to perfectly predict race results with certainty based on training, then we could give out awards before the event even started. But still, every deviation from the ideal circumstances increases the *probability* that you will experience problems.

Injury. If you suffered an injury that hampered training, you should adjust your training to minimize the risk of a reoccurrence. Perhaps more cross-training and core strengthening would have helped, or perhaps your buildup was too rapid. Consulting a coach, trainer, or physical therapist could help you make adjustments to your program.

Pre-Race Taper. Let's move on to you pre-race taper. Did you get enough rest in the weeks, days, and hours before the race? Were you getting over a cold? Jet-lagged? Distracted by work or family problems? All of these factors could have affected your race performance. To the extent that you can control them, you can make changes in your taper in the future.

Uncontrollable Factors. Now, on to race day. Look first at the things outside your control. How was the weather? The ideal temperature for racing is generally thought of as being around 55 degrees Fahrenheit. That's the temperature at which your body finds stasis and feels neither too hot nor too cold once you are warmed up and running. How far off this mark were conditions on your race day? What were the humidity, pollen, and pollution levels? Was it raining or snowing? Hot and sunny? Windy? All these conditions would affect your performance. Warm temperatures can cause dehydration, which can slow you down significantly. Strong sun and glare can wear on you. Cold can make you uncomfortable. You can't change the weather, but you can take all of this into account when you decide where and in what season to race.

How was the support on the course? Were there adequate supplies of water, sports drink, food, and electrolytes? You may decide to bring your own fuel with you next time so that you don't have to rely on the race organizers, or pick a bigger, more established race that could be trusted to nail down details like this.

Perhaps the problem wasn't the availability of fuel and drink, but the amount you took. There's a tendency to think that we have to stop at every aid station on a course, but I look at them like coffee shops—you'll see many of them, but you don't have to stop at each one. When you near an aid station, try to honestly assess if you need anything. Remember to take the weather into account; if it's hot, you may need to pay more attention to fluid replacement. Since we sweat less in cool weather, fluid replacement probably isn't as much of an issue. If you decide that you don't need anything at the aid station, swing wide to avoid slowing runners and keep going.[34]

How was the overall experience? Were there enough spectators and music on the course to motivate you? Did you find the race to be too crowded, or were there so few runners that you found yourself running alone at times? Or maybe you didn't care one way or the other.

Your Running. All of these issues should be considered when you pick your next race. But now let's now consider the part within your control—your running.

If you kept track of your split times, you could analyze where you sped up or slowed down. Be careful to remember anything that could explain anomalies, like any stops at aid stations or Port-a-Jons, or to tie your shoes. After taking that into account, did you run slower during the back half of the race than you did in the first half? If so, how much did you slow down? If it was significant, more than a minute per mile, we need to figure out why.

If the course had more uphills in the second half of the race than the first, then a negative split doesn't necessarily indicate a loss of power. You might have been able to maintain the same

---

34 Exercise physiologists have come to recognize that the risks of dehydration may have been overstated, and the risks of overhydration, called hyponatremia, may be the greater concern. Tim Noakes, *Waterlogged: The Serious Problem of Overhydration in Endurance Sports* (Human Kinetics, 2012).

intensity as in the first half of the race; you just slowed down because of the hills, so your positive split doesn't necessarily mean that you pushed your body past its limit.

Incidentally, you may think that running downhill is easier than running uphill because you can go faster with less effort. That's true, but it comes at a price. The quadriceps muscles on the front of your thighs have to absorb the shock of impact while running and stabilize your leg as you land, and downhill running increases the forces that your quads are trying to control. Downhill running can be fun, but your quads will probably be especially sore for the next couple of days.

If you ran a positive split, and your slowing pace wasn't due to the course or the weather, then you probably pushed your body harder than it was prepared to go. We know this because racers generally don't slow down intentionally; if you slow down, it's because your body simply cannot maintain the pace at which you'd been running.

Simply put, either you didn't train hard enough for the race you planned to run, or you got carried away at the start of the race and ran faster than you had planned. Either way, you will now have to give your body a little more recovery time. Going forward, you can make the necessary adjustments to ensure that you don't make this mistake again. The old saying bears repeating here: train the way you'll race and race the way you've trained.

Your post-race analysis is now complete. You not only have a better idea of what you need to do in the future to improve, but you also have some idea of what your post-race recovery will be over the coming days.

One way of looking at your post-race recovery is to mirror your pre-race taper, but in reverse. So while you slowly scaled back your training as you neared the race, you can slowly ramp up your training in the days and weeks following it.

Another approach is to apply the rule of thumb that says you'll probably need to take one easy day in training for every hard mile you raced. So, you will only need a few days to get back to feeling like your old self after racing a 5K, a week after a 10K, and up to month after a marathon.

You can now adjust those numbers up or down depending on what your race analysis told you about your effort. If you ran a negative split on a flat course, your recovery might be relatively quick. But if you ran on a very hilly course, or ran a positive split, you may need a bit more time. But inevitably, you will recover, and you can start planning your next race.

PLANNING A RACE SCHEDULE

If you followed a healthy post-race recovery plan—refueling and rehydrating as soon as possible right after the race, then slowly building back up your running routine—then you can likely get back out there into a race, or even several, fairly soon.

If you're thinking about running more than one race, you're talking about something new: a race season. Just as every workout should fit into your overall training plan, every race in a season should fit into an overall scheme.

Consider what your goals are for each race you would like to do. Few runners could plan to race at a high level week after week. Still, you may decide to push for a maximum effort in each race that you enter. In that case, you would need to make sure that you fully recover after each effort, build up to another training peak, and then taper for the next big effort. Your race season, then, may not contain many races, but what you sacrifice in quantity, you make up for in quality.

Conversely, you may run all your races at an easy pace, savoring the experience each time. These races would amount to training runs done with hundreds or thousands of other runners. They don't require any special preparation or recovery. Nonetheless, a long race like a half or full marathon can still take a toll on the body, even if done at a slower pace, so you may decide not to participate in too many of these longer races within a given year.

Many runners decide to target one or two key races each year for a very hard effort and use other races as tune-ups. For example, if you are building toward a 10-mile race, you can plan to run several 5Ks or 10Ks beforehand, as long as they are at least a week or more apart from each other and before your big race. As we know, longer races require more recovery, so a 10K or a 10-mile race should be run at least two weeks before a target race.

Here in my hometown of Washington, DC, I get to see elite runners put this strategy into action. Our big springtime racing event is the Cherry Blossom 10-Miler, held annually in early April. It offers significant prize money, but that's not the only thing that attracts elite runners; it usually takes place two weeks before the Boston Marathon. That makes the Cherry Blossom 10-Miler the perfect tune-up race before their big target race.

A race schedule, then, should resemble a good piece of music. There would be a flow to it, with one or more highlights or crescendos. These peaks would be the target races, the ones that matter the most.

But races don't need to be just lead-ups to longer races in a race season. They can also serve other purposes. Shorter-to-middle-distance road races like the 5K and 10K can also be used as a substitute for tempo runs and speed sessions in your training. After all, it's more fun to run with a crowd on race day than to do laps by yourself on a track.

These races can also be used as tests of your fitness throughout the season. If you do a 5K every month during racing season, you would expect your times to improve as you get stronger and faster. If that's not the case, you could tweak your training accordingly to get back on track. Or, instead, if you race faster than you expected, you might raise the difficulty of your training to match your unexpectedly higher fitness level.

ARE YOU IN THE MOOD TO RACE?

In general, you should look forward to the races you've scheduled on your calendar. Some may be more important to you than others—your target races, for example—but they should all, more or less, be events that you get excited about.

If you find that this isn't the case, that racing and even training is starting to feel like a chore, then you should reconsider participating in that race, and perhaps even take a break from hard training.

As long-distance runners, we're used to pushing past our negative thoughts, but sometimes these thoughts indicate a deeper tiredness that we should not ignore. Think of your enthusiasm for running and your risk of injury as being on a continuum. Bouts of burnout and injury are often immediately preceded by a lack of enthusiasm.

This leads back to one of my rules for training and racing: *don't bully your body*. Don't try to force your body through a race or a workout when it honestly tells you that it doesn't want to do it. In my experience, forcing your body to race against its will never turns out well. Instead, partner with your body, and figure out together how and when to race.

This approach might require you to look at your racing schedule a little differently. People use races as a lever to get themselves moving, but no one should treat race schedules as if they are carved in stone. Not even elite athletes. Instead, view them only as options. If you don't dictate a schedule to your body, but instead train smart and let your body tell you if it feels like racing, your chance of sustaining an injury will be much, much lower.

Those are the whys, hows, and whens of road racing. You now know enough to get started and, if you've already been racing, to get more out of it. You know how to prepare for it and how to fit it into your overall training plan.

You might think that's all there is to say about racing. You'd be wrong. The wonderful thing about racing is that it's a puzzle that you can tinker with for a lifetime, trying out new approaches and ideas.

I've been racing for over three decades at this point—a fact that startles me even as I write it—and I'm still trying to figure out how to do it right. As long as I'm racing, that search will continue. I'm forever trying to achieve that perfect race, although I know that perfection is an unachievable goal. Still, I aim to be a little faster and stronger with each race.

Perhaps that's the ultimate attraction of racing. In our fruitless quest for perfection, we aim to become more than who we've been, to achieve something great and timeless. To touch immortality. We try to soar, like Icarus on his false wings, higher and higher.

But, like Icarus, sometimes we come crashing down. In the next chapter we'll tackle the most dreaded running topic: injury.

CHAPTER SEVEN

DEALING WITH RUNNING INJURIES

If running is so good for me, why does it sometimes hurt?

Inevitably, there is that moment. You're in the middle of a good run, and suddenly you feel a twinge. Maybe it's in your hamstring, your knee, or a spot down in your Achilles tendon. But something just sends sparks to your brain. Something is wrong.

You keep running because you're sure that it will work itself out, as these things sometimes do. But this one doesn't. It's there for the rest of your run, and it's still with you later at home. Later, perhaps the next day, you run a few steps to test it, and it flares up again, worse than the day before.

There's no doubt about it now. You're injured.

I try not to pull punches with my clients on this: if you run, you will get injured. That's the reality. Estimates vary because the definition of "injury" varies and many go unreported, but the rate of injury for runners may be as high as 79 percent and is likely around at least 40 percent.[35]

The vast majority of these injuries—around 80 percent—are overuse injuries, which occur when we run too much, too soon, and too fast for our bodies to handle. The leg and the lower back are usually the victims here, with knee injuries being the most common. Looking more closely, we see that connective tissue, or tendons and ligaments, are particularly susceptible to injury. That's because those tissues don't adapt to stress as quickly as muscle, so they can't handle increasing loads as quickly.

Beyond overuse, there are many factors that lead to the possibility of injury. The evidence is often contradictory and inconclusive, but physiology, lifestyle, and activity history all play a role.[36] Because of the range of possibilities, it's hard to predict exactly who will get hurt and when, but we can be sure that somewhere down the road, it will happen. The question, then, is what to do when it does.

RECOGNIZING THE ONSET OF AN INJURY

I had a personal training client once who felt a pain in his chest one day shortly after we had begun working together. Not one

---

35 See, for example, Nicolas Kakouris et al., "A Systematic Review of Running-Related Musculoskeletal Injuries in Runners," *Journal of Sport and Health Science* 10, no. 5 (September 2021): 513–22.

36 Maarten van der Worp et al., "Injuries in Runners: A Systematic Review on Risk Factors and Sex Differences," *PLOS One* 10, no. 2 (February 2015): e0114937.

to take chances, he rushed to the hospital emergency room, fearing that he was suffering a heart attack. The doctors there administered a battery of tests, all of which showed that his heart was functioning normally.

Finally, a doctor asked him if he had just begun exercising. "Yes," he replied. The doctor smiled. "You're just sore," he said. "Go home and rest."

When my client told me this story, he was appropriately sheepish about it, but it illustrated an important point: we need to be able to distinguish ordinary, routine soreness from active injury.

Whenever we stress our bodies with exercise, we create microtears in the muscle fibers of the body parts we used. Our body's response is to create inflammation in the area, which triggers healing. During this healing process, the body re-sculpts the tissue to adapt to the new stress. If you've lifted heavy weights, the muscle will thicken and enable you to generate more power. If you've been running, your body will pack the muscles with additional mitochondria, enabling them to produce more energy so that you can run more miles.

Soreness, then, and even some inflammation are the natural and even desired results of exercise. We push our bodies to create a training stimulus, and our bodies answer with an adaptation response. Some soreness is just an indicator that you've triggered this process, the way that a scrape might sting when you rub it with alcohol.[37]

---

37 Note, however, that this does not mean that if you're not sore, you didn't train hard enough. For a host of reasons, this isn't true, so don't become a soreness junkie.

This process is not instantaneous. Sometimes the soreness doesn't appear until the day after the stimulus, so you may work out on Monday, feel great that night at dinner with your friends, and then feel achy and sore the following day. This is called delayed onset muscle soreness, or DOMS. It's common and entirely normal. It's what happened to my client who misunderstood what he felt when he rushed to the hospital.

But, as with so many things in life, it's possible to have too much of a good thing. If we create more stress than our bodies can handle, we can get hurt. We can think of this process in equation form:

Exercise Stress < Current Level of Fitness = No Improvement/Loss of Fitness

Exercise Stress = Current Level of Fitness = Maintenance of Current Level of Fitness

Exercise Stress > Current Level of Fitness and < Limit of Ability to Adapt = Improvement

Exercise Stress > Limit of Ability to Adapt = Injury

Our goal then is to make sure that we apply exactly the right amount of stress on our muscles to exceed our current level of fitness, but only enough to trigger improvement, not an injury.

Maybe you'll be the one who will finally get this right all the time. I'll be rooting for you. More likely, though, you will, like the rest of us, get it right most of the time but occasionally get it wrong. There are warning signs to look for that would tell you when you've stepped over this line:

- Pain that gets worse, not better, over the course of several days
- Sharp, specific pain, instead of overall soreness
- Visible swelling

If you're experiencing any of these signs, you're probably injured. This isn't the end of the world, however, especially if you can recognize the situation clearly and respond appropriately. Usually, this happens in steps. Sometimes the issue isn't an injury, but an illness. The rule for training and racing through routine sickness is that you can run through congestion—and in fact running might make you feel better—but stop completely if you have a fever, aches, or a sore throat. Let your body concentrate its resources on getting better.

STAGES OF BEING INJURED

Denial is usually the first stage of being injured. We think that whatever pain we feel while running will work itself out. Sometimes it does, but when it persists, we think it will certainly be better the following day. This might lead to the bargaining phase, where we promise ourselves a day off, or that we'll ice the affected area, in the belief that with just a little attention we'll be good as new. Sometimes this works, but when it doesn't, we have to face the truth.

This is a crucial moment. You've recognized that you have an injury. What you do next will determine whether you recover quickly and get back to running, or whether you'll be laid up for weeks or more.

Acceptance is most often the next phase. In the example that opened this chapter, we imagined this exact scenario. At this stage, it's common for many of us to grumble and wallow in a bit of self-pity. We feel like we're the only ones who are suffering, especially when we see so many other happy runners cruising the trails and streets. A friend of mine told me that when she's injured, she curses them all.

Of course, it's never *only* us. It's just the moment when it *is* us. As tempting as it is to think of an injury as something that happened *to* us, like being hit by a bolt of lightning, the truth is that it's almost always the result of something that we did to ourselves. As we discussed earlier, the culprit is most often overtraining.

Once we recognize this fact, we can see an injury not just as a pain that keeps us from doing what we want, but as a form of communication from our body. In a very crude way, our body is telling us that we are doing something wrong in training, and it wants us to stop.

In this sense, I think of the body like a crying baby. It's telling us that it's unhappy, but it lacks the ability to be specific. We have to figure it out for ourselves. And just as it would do no good to get angry with or resentful toward a crying baby, there's no point either in being angry with our injured body. If we figure out what the problem is and fix it, the crying will stop.

Sometimes the cause of our injury is obvious, like when we add a new element to our training. If you write down your workouts in a logbook, this will be easy to spot. Perhaps you increased your weekly mileage or your long run too quickly, or you eliminated a rest day. Whatever change you made, it would be a good bet that your body didn't like it, and it would appreciate it if you took a more measured approach in the future.

GHOST INJURIES

When is an injury not an injury? When it's a ghost injury.

A common phenomenon that runners experience during the taper phase of their race preparation is the sudden appearance of new aches and pains. This can be confusing because this should be the easiest phase of training. If our body seemed fine earlier, during the hardest part of training, why is it complaining now? This can be especially upsetting because the race is only a few weeks or even days away, and there's precious little time to deal with an injury.

To all appearances, these aches and pains—a sore knee, a tender hamstring, an achy Achilles tendon—seem to be serious injuries. They both are and are not.

What you feel is not a figment of your imagination. You do have these aches and pains. But they might not be indicators of a serious underlying injury. Instead, they might just be soreness that your body is dealing with now that the stress of heavy training is over.

Look at it like this: imagine that you've been feeding a baby, but the baby is fighting you because he hates strained peas. He knocks a spoonful to the floor, but you'll deal with that later. Right now, you've got to focus on getting through this feeding.

So, too, with your body. When your body is handling the heavy load of training, it doesn't have the time or ability to deal with little issues that come up. It will deal with those later.

Remember: your body has evolved to hunt and forage for food and to avoid becoming food. It doesn't think that your movements might just be for recreation and competition. Every time that you ask it to move, it thinks that your life might be on the line. That's why your body will find a way to move when you're injured, even if it might put other body parts at risk. Sometimes this requires your body to ignore less serious issues. It does this in the moment by flooding your system with adrenaline and endorphins, which gives you a burst of energy and masks little problems that might distract you from fighting for your life. It also puts some aches or pains on the back burner.

When the training load is reduced—or, in your body's point of view, when the crisis is over—your body may unpack all the little issues that it had put aside and, in our analogy, clean up the floor. Don't stress over it. The aches and pains are real, but probably not as serious as you fear. Stretch, ice, and rest as needed, but don't worry excessively about it. In all likelihood, your body will resolve these issues quickly, and you'll be fine on race day.

Taking action is the next and final phase of dealing with an injury. The first thing I recommend doing after you've realized and accepted that you have an injury is to back off from running. That might sound obvious, but for many of us who really, *really* don't want to stop, we think that cutting back a little will do the trick. But if your body is telling you that it is really unhappy, you should listen to that and shut things down until you figure out the problem.

We would do well at this point to remember our earlier discussion about being smarter than we are brave. The question is not whether we are tough enough to run even while hurt; the question is whether we can be smart enough, and disciplined enough, to do what our body needs us to do instead of what we'd like to do.

One of the toughest parts about pausing your running, at least for me, is dealing with the resulting emotional fallout. Since so much of who I am is defined by my running, I've felt that if I'm not running, I'm no longer who I thought I was. I end up feeling a bit like a fraud.

This mindset is a serious mistake. Running is something we do, something that has added greatly to our lives in so many ways, but we should never forget that it is not all of who we are. We have lives apart from running. Sometimes it takes an injury to remember that.

After you stop doing the thing that probably triggered your injury, the next steps usually include some combination of resting, icing, stretching, and strengthening. Rest to remove the stimulus that caused the problem; ice to bring down the excessive inflammation; stretching to relieve pressure caused by lack of flexibility; and strengthening exercises to eliminate any weakness in the chain of movement that may have contributed to, or even caused, the strain in the first place.

You shouldn't feel like you are all alone on this journey back to health. I firmly believe that every runner should have a team of experts behind them to keep them running. Think of yourself as a race car, and your support team as the pit crew. No race car driver would ever consider getting out of his car to refuel, change the tires, or take care of any mechanical issues that have come up. You should not treat your body with any less care and attention.

COLLECTING YOUR INJURY SUPPORT TEAM

We talked earlier about investing in a coach to help improve your running. Now we should focus on collecting your medical team.

Finding a good doctor is like finding a good car mechanic or home improvement contractor; once you've found someone knowledgeable whom you can trust, you should hold on to them tightly. Aim for a doctor and therapists who won't just say, "Don't do that," but who will instead say, "Here's what you need to do so you can get back to doing the thing you love."

While it's not essential that your medical team be composed of people who run, I've found that this is usually the best scenario. If your doctors and therapists are runners, they understand how you feel and how important it is to you to get back on the roads as soon as possible.

Over the course of my running life, I've been treated by many doctors, and the report card is mixed. I've respected them all and have appreciated their work, but I've felt that some of them were partners in helping me get back to running and others, well, not so much.

Orthopedists in particular have presented a challenge. I've had several who have told me how awful running is for my body. Interestingly, they do this at the same time that they compliment me on my great overall fitness, leaving me wondering how they think I've attained that fitness if not by running. Still, the most positive opinion about running that I've ever gotten from an orthopedist is this: "Running is the worst thing that you could do, except for not running."

I don't dislike orthopedists; I deeply respect their expertise and the help many of them have given me over the years. I even understand their dislike of running. The reason for this occurred to me once in a flash. The problem is that all the runners they meet in their practice are hurt, so they must naturally start to think that all running hurts. With this in mind, I've wondered whether I should make an appointment with an orthopedist when I'm feeling fine, which is most of the time, just to let them know that I'm running happy and injury-free.

As a running patient—really, as a patient in any circumstance—I'm a firm believer in assuming an active role in this process. Ask your doctor any and all questions that occur to you; you are not wasting their time, and you have every right to do so.

You may, on occasion, need to move from doctor to doctor until you find the one who can help you. I once had a pain in my foot that was misdiagnosed as plantar fasciitis (PF), an inflammation of the connective tissue on the sole of the foot. I was suspicious, since my symptoms did not fully square up with the typical signs of PF, but I gamely followed the doctor's advice, and the advice of the next doctor to treat me, and the one after that. I endured wearing a night boot, doing strengthening exercises, and getting a cortisone shot, all to no avail. Then, finally, a doctor diagnosed my problem as originating not in my foot, but in my ankle, which was not moving properly on foot-strike.

He did some manipulations of my ankle bones to restore full range of motion, and magically, my pain disappeared.

The takeaway from this story is that even good doctors can sometimes misdiagnose a problem. I don't believe that pain occurs randomly; there is a reason for every pain that you feel. Your body may not be very articulate in explaining what the problem is, but it is sending you a true message nonetheless. If one doctor doesn't seem to be able to figure it out, move on to the next one. Eventually, someone should come up with the right answer.

MEDICAL SPECIALISTS

A general practitioner might be able to help you with some of your running problems, but I've found it more useful to consult with specialists. A nonexhaustive list of the experts that you should have on your team could include the following:

- **Orthopedist**—This is the go-to doctor for all sports injuries. If your hip or knee is troubling you, this is the doctor for you.
- **Podiatrist**—Treats all ankle and foot injuries.
- **Physical Therapists**—These practitioners try to correct a faulty motor pattern or a muscle strength imbalance. They can also usually perform a detailed gait analysis.
- **Chiropractor**—Some pain that we experience is caused by a misalignment of the hips and spine. When this is the issue, a

chiropractor can often return us to health relatively quickly.

- **Nutritionist**—Running can stress your gastrointestinal system, and finding out what our bodies can and cannot tolerate—on a regular basis or on race day—can be a difficult task. Coaches may be able to offer general advice, but they are not qualified to give detailed nutritional advice.

Once you've built up your circle of medical practitioners, you should make use of them. This is probably something that most of us need to work on. Our default setting seems to be that while we may complain about our aches or pains, we expect them to simply go away on their own. It's only after the ache or pain gets much, much worse that we seek help.

I want to put an end to that approach. Instead of making a doctor's visit the last resort, let's make it the first option, because if you think something is wrong, it probably is. The sooner you get it properly diagnosed, the sooner you will get it resolved. Your running buddies, your neighborhood running-store owner, and your barista may all have great advice, but none of them are doctors. Besides, you (hopefully!) have medical insurance that you pay for—so use it. In all likelihood, the first available appointment is probably a week or more away, and if your issue resolves over the next few days, you could always cancel that appointment. But if you wait a week and it still bothers you, you will have to wait yet another week to see a doctor.

Not only should you make use of your medical team, you should also share their contact information with your friends the way you would share restaurant recommendations. Offer up your own good experiences to your friends and ask for theirs. You can never have too many doctors that you can rely on. It's not just good karma; your doctors will appreciate the referrals, and they might be inclined to make space for you in their packed schedules when you most need it.

STICKING WITH YOUR TREATMENT PLAN

When we are injured, we tend to follow the recovery plan that our doctor recommends to the letter. We ice, massage, manipulate, stretch, and work the area exactly as instructed because we trust our doctors—or we try to—and if following their advice will make us healthy again, then doing as we're told is a small price to pay.

But then a funny thing happens. We start to feel better. As our sense of panic begins to recede and we dare to run again, we forget to do the things our doctor told us to do to get and stay healthy. It all doesn't seem so urgent anymore. If we're pressed for time, we promise ourselves to do it later, and then later never seems to come. And then—not all the time, but at least sometimes—the pain returns, and we're back at square one. Be smart and learn this lesson once.

THE ROAD BACK

My first attempt at running a marathon ended before I even arrived at the starting line. After successfully completing my training, I was only a week away from the race when I went for a trail run with my roommate. A few miles into the run, I took a bad step and twisted my ankle on a rock. Now I would have gone straight home to treat the sprain, but back then I was sure that all I needed to do was to keep running and the pain would go away. It did not. Instead, I ended up in the emergency room, and then on crutches. There would be no marathon for me that year.

There's a lesson in there, to be sure, but that's not why I'm telling you this story. It's what happened next that should interest us now. Instead of letting my ankle heal and slowly getting back to running, I kept rushing my recovery and reinjuring it. That strategy turned what should have been a three- or four-week layoff into a six-month hiatus.

The lesson here is clear: don't rush your return. But that lesson is actually made up of five separate lessons about the road to injury recovery:

Remember your history. The number one risk factor for an injury is having had that injury before. You can't change the past, but you can influence the future. Be extra careful to avoid whatever caused your injury earlier, and as we just discussed, be sure to continue the regimen that brought you back to health.

Build back up gradually and consider possible limits. Don't try to get your fitness back all at once. It might be tempting to jump up to long miles as soon as possible in order to catch up to where your training plan says you should be, but that might just put you back on the injured reserve list.

Aim to close the gap slowly, week by week. The rule of thumb is to increase the long run and the weekly total mileage by no more than 10 percent week to week; this ensures that your body has only a manageable amount of stress to deal with. This game of catch-up could take a month or more, so be patient.

Keep in mind also that we all have a comfort zone for mileage, and what's safe for someone else might not be safe for you. Just because your friend set a personal record in the marathon after logging 80-mile weeks in training doesn't mean their plan will work for you. With time, you'll find what combination of training stimuli works best for you. This is hard-earned knowledge. Don't ignore it.

Consider using cross-training to speed up your recovery. Your heart and lungs don't care what you choose to do to improve your health, so you can add nonimpact cross-training to supplement your running. Running simulators, like the elliptical machine or pool-running, can get you ready for road running, and cycling helps by targeting muscles that are not primarily strengthened by running, such as the quadriceps muscles of the front of the leg. By strengthening these muscles, you actually reduce the risk of injury in the future.

Work the core. This has become a favorite catchphrase of our exercise culture, but it's true: a weak core is often the culprit behind injury. That's because weakness in the core—defined as all the muscles from mid-thigh to the bottom of the ribcage, front, back, and sides—can compromise running form. This results in some muscles not doing their job, while others get overloaded. Take a class or talk with a trainer about improving your core strength, but just get it done. It won't take long, and doing this just twice a week for 15 minutes or so will make a real difference.

Take a break. Remember our earlier lesson: if you're unusually tired and uninspired before a particular run, chances are that your body is stressed, and a stressed body is more susceptible to injury. Take a day off.

Don't rush your readiness to race. Looking back over the years, I can easily see a pattern to my injuries and failed races: whenever I focused on my race date to guide my training, rather than relying on how my body felt, I ran into problems. The lesson for us is to keep our race date and training plan in mind, but not to let it dictate our training. We need to give paramount importance to what our bodies tell us. If this puts competing in a particular race in jeopardy, so be it. No race is worth getting hurt.

TURNING LEMONS INTO A LEMONADE-FLAVORED SPORTS DRINK

It's hard to think of an injury as a good thing; there's no real upside to being hurt. Still, having an injury can open the door to changing our routine and lifestyle in a way that will leave us better off in the long run.

For guidance in this approach, I take as my mantra the Chinese word for "crisis": *weiji*. That word is made up of two characters, 危机 in simplified Chinese and 危機 in traditional Chinese. The first character means danger, and the second, opportunity.[38] The spirit of *weiji* is to find new possibilities for progress when things go wrong.

---

38 Some linguists have called this translation incorrect, but that doesn't really matter to me. I care less about the word than I do on the meaning that I take from my understanding of it, so if this isn't what it really means, I feel it's what it *should* mean, at least for us.

An example of this in action is a story I've heard about the great boxer Larry Holmes, who was the heavyweight champion of the world back in the 1980s. Early in his career he hurt his right hand, a devastating injury for the right-handed fighter. Nevertheless, instead of simply doing nothing while he waited for his hand to heal, he kept going to the gym to work on the only thing still available to him: his left hand. He ended up developing one of the most formidable left jabs in the history of the sport.

The takeaway is that by thinking creatively, we can use the downtime forced on us by an injury to lay the groundwork for being an even healthier, more injury-resistant runner when we get back on the roads. By focusing on something other than how much we resent not being able to run, we can begin to think positively about our situation.

With that in mind, think of ways that you could improve your health and fitness during this hiatus. Perhaps you could work on improving your diet or on building core strength and flexibility. You might be able to work on different forms of cross-training. Indeed, many of the alternate exercise routines that I developed while injured later became part of my regular program when I got back to running.

LEARN TO TRUST AGAIN

Whether we realize it or not, we are all involved in a relationship with our bodies. Like all relationships, it is based on trust, and when trust is broken, it takes time for that breach to heal.

For your body, that breach occurred when you subjected it to stress that it could not handle. Your body responded as best it could, perhaps by changing its movement patterns and relying on other muscles to get the job done, because getting it done was what you asked it to do. This put great stress on your body, which resulted in the injury itself and in spasms in the surrounding muscles, which your body activated to protect the injured tissue. This is why doctors often prescribe not only anti-inflammatories to injured athletes but muscle relaxers as well. Before healing can fully take place, the body has to calm down from the stress that *you* placed on it. Massage and stretching can help with this process, too.

Sometimes physical therapy is required to re-establish normal movement patterns. When you were injured, your body learned to move in a different, inefficient, and potentially harmful way to protect the injured tissue. That's what limping is really all about, for example. Often, proper movement returns as soon as healing is complete, but sometimes the body has to be coaxed back to moving correctly. This takes time and multiple visits to a physical therapist. Eventually, your body will trust in you again and will move as it should.

You, too, need to trust again. As animals, we naturally try to avoid pain, and the memory of running in pain can cause deeper trauma and anxiety than you might at first realize. After recovering from an injury, you may hesitate to run, avoiding hard workouts even after you've been cleared to do them. You've lost faith in your body's ability to run hard without pain.

For both you and your body, trust will be restored incrementally with each pain-free run. Eventually, both of you will believe in your ability to run hard without pain, and you will rediscover the joy that you had for running before you became injured. Once this two-way trust is back, you could register for your next race.

TO PROTECT AND SERVE ONESELF

There have been too many times when I was reckless with my running. I trained through injury, raced when I ought not have, and sometimes failed to properly feed and hydrate my body. I always thought that I would weather these thoughtless moments, and that everything would be fine as long as I was aware of the risks. Often, it all worked out.

But sometimes I had to pay the price for being reckless. I've had layoffs from injury, and uninspired training and racing. I sometimes did things that made me not like running quite as much. I should have been more protective of my running. After all, much as I would like to believe that I have a bottomless pit of running, I know people who can no longer run as often, as far, or as fast as they once were able to, or even run at all. We can tell ourselves that we won't end up like that, but I'd bet that those people thought that very same thing.

I'm reminded about the wisdom of the legendary Kenyan-American miler and Olympian Bernard Lagat, who ran competitively well into his 40s, an age when most elite runners were telling old racing stories from their comfy armchairs. Lagat attributed his longevity to completely shutting down his training for a month every year after his racing season was over. This was how he protected himself.

I'm not suggesting that we should avoid striving for running excellence. What I am saying is that we should take a mature, responsible approach to running, in which hard work, dedication, determination, and clear-eyed reason guide us in equal measure to achieving our goals. We just have to aim to do so with as many safeguards in place as possible.

THE GIFT OF INJURY

It's hard to think of an injury as being a good thing. I'm not going to try to convince you otherwise. But that's not the same as saying that there is absolutely no value to being injured.

As we discussed earlier, an injury can present an opportunity to add new and important elements to your training, filling gaps that have kept you from becoming a more injury-resistant, efficient, and powerful runner.

An injury can also give you time to reconnect with friends and family. You might discover that they missed you when you were off on a long run every Sunday morning. It can give you time to catch up on old hobbies or create new ones. You'll have more time to read books, see movies, and maybe even stay up late. As your injury heals, other little aches and pains may disappear as well, now that you've given your entire body a chance to rest.

All this is true, and yet none of it seems to me to be especially compelling. But when I think of an injury as being a gift,

I'm thinking about something a bit deeper, a bit more philo-sophical.

Every semester, I take the group from the running class that I instruct on a special run. We go up Massachusetts Avenue on a stretch that's known as Embassy Row. It's an uphill run, but we distract ourselves by ticking off the different embassies as we pass them: Ireland, India, Japan, France, Brazil, and Britain.

Across the street, on the north side, is the embassy of South Africa. When I was in college, I came down from New York with a busload of people to protest apartheid in front of that embassy and to demand the release of Nelson Mandela from prison. Now, as we run past, I point out to my students the statue of Nelson Mandela, raising his fist skyward in defiance of his captors and in celebration of the victory over oppression and hate. Despite all the chaos in the world, passing this statue reminds me of the change I have witnessed in my own lifetime.

I bring my class to a stop a short distance farther on and lead them off the sidewalk into a small memorial park dedicated to the Lebanese poet Khalil Gibran. There is a bronze bas-relief sculpture of Gibran by the entrance, and in the center is a star-shaped fountain filled with black river stones, surrounded by a circular limestone bench featuring engraved lines of his poetry.

I gather the class around one particular bench, and I read aloud the quote engraved there: "Do not the spirits who dwell in the ether envy man his pain?"

I ask them for their thoughts on this quote, but this is a running class, and after a few miles of running uphill, inter-preting a line of poetry might be bit much for them. So I offer mine.

I tell them that Gibran is reminding us that spirits are unfeeling, knowing neither joy nor sorrow, and long to feel something, *anything*, even the unhappiness that was sometimes a part of being alive.

As a runner, I tell them, when I read those words, I am reminded of the times when I have been injured, when my running shoes lay untouched by the front door, waiting like a pet dog to be taken outside. On those days, have longed for even the worst of my runs—those days when my legs felt like lead and all the roads felt like they're uphill. When the miracle finally occurred and I could run again, I tried to recall that feeling, and to never take a run—*any* run—for granted.

My students usually nod appreciatively, but they are young, and most of them don't yet have the life experience to really understand what I'm trying to tell them. But if they remember this conversation, someday they will.

In the end, Gibran's words are just like those I had spotted once on a sign held up by a spectator during a race: "Someday you will not be able to do this. Today is not that day."

If, then, every injury is a reminder of our mortality, then every recovery should be a celebration, the yin to injury's yang. Appreciate the gift, take whatever lessons your body is trying to tell you, and then try like hell not to get injured again.

SPRINTING TO THE FINISH

It's one of the most exciting moments in all of sports. Two highly trained athletes racing neck-and-neck to the finish line, the distance between them seemingly thinner than a hair's width. Effort and pain are etched on their faces as they give every last bit of energy and will that they have left to win the race.

Very few runners will experience the thrill of giving an all-out effort to win a race, but many runners still choose to sprint to the finish line, even if the winner has already crossed long before. Some are trying to beat their friends or a stranger who they've randomly picked as their rival for the moment. Others just get motivated by the roar of the crowd, while a few are pushing themselves to get in just under the wire for a new personal record or even a Boston qualifier.[39]

Earlier we discussed a negative split, where you run the second half of a race faster than the first. Generally, among the best runners, this drop is only a handful of seconds. Overall, the fastest mile is not so dramatically different from the slowest mile.

Holding a steady pace with a slight negative split is the most efficient way to race. When I see a slower runner sprinting to the finish, I think that they've made a mistake in either their planning or their racing.

Sprinting at the end of a long-distance race also raises the risk of injury. That's why I raise this topic now. After running for hours, fatigue sets in and our form begins to break down. Sprinting at

---

39 The Boston Marathon is one of the very few races that accepts only runners who have met their qualifying standards in a previous marathon. Getting a Boston qualifier, or "BQ," as they're known, is the Holy Grail of distance running.

this point opens the door to a possible strain or tear.

I also have a theory about how sprinting ties in with runner mortality. While it's extremely rare to die during a marathon, when it does happen, it tends to be near, at, or just past the finish line. I believe several factors can contribute to this.

First, there is no way to fully simulate the stress of a marathon in the lab, so some runners race without knowing that they have a heart abnormality. Second, many of the sports gels that marathoners commonly use are loaded with caffeine, making each gel the equivalent of one or two cups of coffee. If a runner takes four to six gels during a race, which is not unusual, it would be like drinking ten or so cups of coffee. All that caffeine raises the risk of a cardiac event. On top of these circumstances, add the stress of a finish-line sprint, and you have a perfect storm of risk factors to possibly explain a runner's death.

Of course, there's no way to prove this because we'll probably never know those kinds of details about a runner after the fact. And yes, there are still all those great reasons to sprint. But I would ask you if finishing just a little faster is worth a layoff—or worse—because of an injury. Perhaps to you it is. Fair enough. Just be sure that you understand the risks involved and make an informed decision. As we discussed earlier, *be purposeful*.

CHAPTER EIGHT

AGING AND RUNNING

The time you won your town the race
We chaired you through the market-place;
Man and boy stood cheering by,
And home we brought you shoulder-high.
Today, the road all runners come,
Shoulder-high we bring you home,
And set you at your threshold down,
Townsman of a stiller town.
Smart lad, to slip betimes away
From fields where glory does not stay,
And early though the laurel grows
It withers quicker than the rose.

Excerpt from "To an Athlete Dying Young,"
by A. E. Housman[40]

---

40 A. E. Housman, *A Shropshire Lad*, 1896.

Ours is a culture that celebrates the beauty, power, and speed of youth, but Time is a thief who eventually steals those attributes from us all. For runners, this is glaringly apparent. In other sports you face an opponent, but in running, the opponent is Time itself, and it never lies, it never falters, and it never loses.

At first, we may dismiss the evidence of our decline as only an aberration. After a subpar performance, we tell ourselves that all we need to do is get a good night's sleep, or train a little harder, and speed will return to our legs like a dog returning at the master's call.

Except that it doesn't. Harder training only brings more soreness and slower times, and maybe even an injury. More sleep and better nutrition don't do the trick either. Grudgingly, we admit the truth. We are not the runner we used to be.

For some people, this causes a seismic shift in their running. I have a friend who was a very strong marathoner, but he gave up running marathons as soon as he could no longer match his best times. For him, there was no point to racing if he couldn't be his best.

Then there's Bill Rodgers, one of the finest marathoners that the United States has ever produced. In the late 1970s and early 1980s, Rodgers won both the Boston Marathon and the New York City Marathon *four times each*. Now, over four decades later, Boston Billy is far behind the lead pack. Still, he's out there running, not expecting to win, but no doubt expecting to push himself to do his best.

So who's right? Both of them, of course. But if you enjoy running, and plan to do it throughout your life, you're going to have to figure out a way to come to terms with getting older.

WHAT IS OLD?

Conventional wisdom holds that old is generally 15 years more than whatever your age is at a given moment. In other words, the concept of old is a moving target and relative to your own situation.

There are also different types of old. In running, when a coach asks you for your age, he may not be asking how old *you* are; he might be asking how old your *legs* are. If you're new to running, you may be old according to your birth certificate, but young when it comes to endurance sports. That's the difference between *chronological age* and *training age*. A runner with young legs can expect that their fastest race times are ahead of them, regardless of how old they are.

But eventually there's no getting around it. Aging brings a diminishment of fitness, and in the world of sports performance, old comes quickly. In general, our bodies reach their peaks for speed and power somewhere in the early to mid 20s. After that, we lose up to 10 percent of our speed and power per decade until we hit our 70s, at which point there's usually a steeper decline in athletic performance.[41]

That might sound depressing, but we need to remember two important facts: First, there's a difference between an athlete's *potential* and their *actual* fitness. And second, exercise at any age can trigger improvements in strength and speed.

To see how this plays out, take a look at the chart below. The vertical axis marks fitness, while the horizontal axis represents age. You'll see two arcs on this chart: segments A-B and C-D.

---

41 These numbers vary a bit depending on the demands of the sport being examined and the gender of the athlete.

You'll notice that while these two segments both roughly describe a peaking arc, they don't track together perfectly. Segment A-B shows us an athlete's potential fitness over their lifetime. Segment C-D, however, shows this athlete's actual fitness. Segment C-D is always below A-B because only very highly trained athletes come close to matching their potential at any time in their careers.[42] But if you look closely, you'll see that segment C-D actually rises up toward the right side of the chart when segment A-B is in decline.

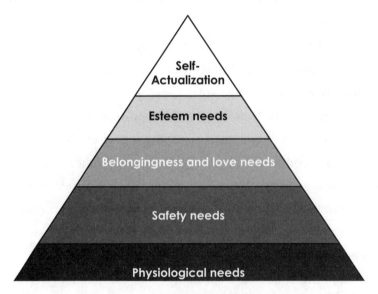

To understand what's happening here, let's invent a story for this athlete, whom we'll call Allison. Allison was not much of an athlete in her 20s, when her body was reaching its highest potential level for speed and power, but some years later, after Allison had worked hard to achieve success in her career, she realized that she had gained some weight, and that she couldn't

---

42 This is always the case, to a greater or lesser degree, as our actual fitness could not logically ever exceed our potential fitness.

climb stairs without getting winded. Allison had gotten out of shape.

With her 40th birthday looming ahead, Allison decided to do something about this. She joined a gym, began working out, and started running with a group three times a week. Slowly, she shed the excess weight and started climbing stairs two at a time. She felt better than she had in years.

Let's now look again at the chart. You'll notice that there is a gray shaded area between the two segments. This represents the difference at any moment in time between Allison's potential fitness and her actual fitness. When she was in her 20s the gap between her potential and actual fitness was at its peak, but by age 40, that gap had shrunk to its smallest size yet as an adult, and was still improving. As Allison's potential fitness declined, her actual fitness had improved, and by age 40, she was actually in the best shape of her life.

This scenario roughly describes the life experience of many runners. While they might have been faster and stronger had they begun running earlier in their lives, they still enjoyed the benefits of running when they finally began training later in life. For them, aging didn't bring decline, despite what segment A-B would have predicted. Because they changed their lifestyle, aging brought them better health.

THE REMARKABLE FAUJA SINGH

For an extreme example of the difference between potential and actual fitness, consider the case of Fauja Singh.

As I write these words, Mr. Singh is 112 years old. Born a sickly child in Punjab in 1911, he took up running as a young man, but gave it up in the 1940s after the bloody partition of India. After suffering the loss of his wife and two children in the 1990s, Mr. Singh emigrated to England to be with one of his sons, and there he returned to running.

At age 89 he ran in his first race, the London Marathon. At age 94 he set a world record in his age group in the marathon, and at age 100 he set eight world age group records in a single track meet in Canada. Shortly after, he finished the Toronto Waterfront Marathon in 8 hours and 11 minutes.

Mr. Singh continued to race until 2013, when he announced his retirement from competitive running, though he continued to run for health and pleasure. By 2023 he was no longer running, although he still attended running events to cheer on competitors.

Clearly, Mr. Singh is a gifted athlete and is in a category all his own. When his race times are analyzed using an age-graded race calculator, his effort in relation to his peer group makes him the fastest marathoner by far who ever lived.

WHAT HAPPENS WHEN WE AGE?

At some point, of course, we're old in any way you look at it, chronologically or by training years. The improvements we made to our bodies top out and begin to decline. Just as running causes specific changes in the body on the way up, aging creates specific changes in our bodies as well. These effects include the following:

- **Lower VO₂ Max.** VO_2 max represents the amount of oxygen that your lungs can deliver to your body. Because oxygen is like fuel for your muscles, your VO_2 max is a good measurement of cardiovascular fitness. As we age, our ability to push oxygen into our working muscles declines, meaning that our ability to sustain hard physical efforts over time also declines.
- **Slower Recovery.** Our bodies produce human growth hormone while we sleep to trigger the repair of damaged tissue, but as we age, we produce less and less of this substance, meaning that our muscles don't recover as quickly after hard workouts as they used to.
- **Loss of Muscle Mass.** Another side effect of diminishing production of human growth hormone is that we cannot build or maintain the amount of muscle mass that we had—or could have had—when we were younger.
- **Reduced Bone Density.** This raises the risk of osteoporosis and stress fractures.
- **Reduced Heart Efficiency.** Our maximum heart rate— the level at which we can spike our beats per minute

when we work hard—slowly diminishes as we age. A lower heart rate means less oxygen and nutrients can be delivered to muscles during exercise, which reduces performance.

- **Loss of Flexibility.** Chemical changes in our tendons lead to stiffness and reduced range of motion.

The combined effect of all these factors is that as we get older, we cannot train as regularly or as hard as we might have when we were younger. This is when the reality of aging sets in. We can no longer rely on the hope that we could get back to the way we used to be with a little bit more effort. As we get older, more exercise at some point doesn't mean more fitness; instead, it just means more problems.

Still, there's some good news. While we cannot completely avoid the effects of aging, we can slow it down with training. Running will help us maintain as much cardiovascular fitness, balance, and strength as possible. To put it bluntly, the only thing worse than aging as a runner is aging as a nonrunner. But to be a senior athlete requires us to begin approaching our training and racing differently.

YOUR EVOLVING RELATIONSHIP WITH YOUR BODY

We've said earlier that a good way to view your body is to think of it as a roommate or close friend with whom you share space. You have a relationship with your body, and over the years, you've experienced many things together. You've taken your first steps as a runner, perhaps competed in races, and come through injuries.

Now, as both of you enter a new phase of your lives together, you will have to adjust the way you think of your body. Don't think of these as rules; these are more like suggestions and considerations.

LISTEN TO YOUR BODY

This is always a good idea, but especially now, because as we age, our margin for error shrinks. We can't just shrug off bad training and racing decisions now as easily as we did when we were younger, when all we needed was a day or two of rest to emerge good as new. Now, ignoring any warning signs from our body can lead to an injury and a layoff from running.

So what does listening to your body look like? It begins by honestly acknowledging signals that your body is giving you. A little soreness isn't just something to run through, and a nagging pain isn't something that we can just assume will go away. Assess how you feel every day, on every run, and take note of anything that seems out of the ordinary.

LET YOUR BODY DECIDE

Your job doesn't end with listening to your body; you need to respond with action. If something seems wrong, take a day off. If the problem persists another day, make an appointment with your doctor. Trust in your body and don't overrule what it tells you.

REMEMBER THAT ACCEPTING CERTAIN LIMITS IS A STRENGTH, NOT A WEAKNESS

A disciplined runner is not someone who can deal with pain; it's someone who can do the oftentimes difficult work of avoiding pain. Being a senior runner should not just be about age; it should be about wisdom. After years of running, you should know how to partner with your body. Don't turn your partnership into a dictatorship. As in any relationship, listening is usually more important than talking, and sometimes not taking action—not training, not racing—is the hardest thing to do. I've had clients who were dedicated enough to train hard, but who were not dedicated enough to back off when they were supposed to. Learn to be dedicated in the best ways.

DON'T BE AFRAID TO PUSH

If everything you just read leads you to believe that I think older runners should ease into gentle Sunday jogs, you'd be dead wrong. Fitness comes from discomfort; do not be afraid to push your body just because you're older. In fact, this is when pushing harder is the most important. Just be sure to do it intelligently. Recognize that discomfort is not the same thing as pain. Listen to your body, but when your body does not give you any good reason to back off, like an ache or pain, prepare to push hard.

This is the key to maintaining speed as we age. One of the main reasons runners slow down as they get older is that they stop running fast. Perhaps it's just not as much fun as it used to be, or they've read that they should slow down as they age. But the simple truth is that being an older runner is, in this regard, the same as being a younger runner: to get faster we need to run faster. Don't be afraid to do that when the conditions are right.

HAVE A PREPARATION AND RECOVERY PLAN

When I began running, my pre-run routine was to get out of bed, get dressed, and go out the door. My post-run routine was a quick shower.

My days look very different now. As an older athlete, I begin every day with at least a short warm-up and some stretching or yoga, and I do some run-specific warm-ups before I head out the door. I finish my workouts with more stretching and often foam rolling as well. At first, I did these things reluctantly and with resentment, but over the months and years, I've come to enjoy them. I can now even see their value independently, not just as tools to keep me running. Best of all, I can say that I now have better balance and flexibility than I ever did when I was younger.

LOOK FORWARD, NOT BACK

A few years ago, I found myself feeling anxious about an upcoming get-together. I was planning to meet up with a pack of my former running buddies whom I had not seen in years. Recalling how fast many of them were, I worried that I would be ashamed of my current state of running. I even considered not going to the event at all.

I needn't have worried. While it was true that I wasn't the runner that I had used to be, neither were they. Some had even given up running entirely. My place among my peers was at least as good as it had been years ago, and perhaps now even better.

My mistake was in assuming that as I aged, everyone else was living in a bubble, eternally young, fast, and strong. Ridiculous, I know, but I was locked into looking backward, and that's what my brain told me I would see.

The great Czech Olympic champion Emil Zátopek once said, "Don't look back. You're not going that way." That's as good advice for running and life as I've ever heard. While it's wonderful to recall past achievements, we need to detach from them. That runner is not who we are now, and that's fine, because with a little work, we can be a strong, competitive runner in our current age group.

Don't compete with your past. That's not a race you could ever win.

ENJOY THE MOMENT

We talked earlier about being grateful for even our worst training days, and this is doubly true for older runners. If we spend all our time regretting that we're not 20 years old anymore, we lose the opportunity to enjoy the moment we're in and to celebrate the kind of runner we are now.

Here's a reality check for you: no matter how slow you are right now, there will come a day when you look back and wish that you could be this fast again, or be able to run at all. Don't wait for that to happen before you appreciate who you are right now.

Consider the legendary Boston Marathon champion Johnny Kelley. Born in Medford, Massachusetts, in 1907, Kelley represented the US in the marathon in the Olympics, in 1936 and 1948, and won the Boston Marathon twice, in 1935 and 1945. He placed second in the Boston Marathon another seven times. In fact, from 1934 to 1950 he placed in the top five in the Boston Marathon 15 times.

But it's not just these great accomplishments that Kelley is remembered for. He went on to compete in the Boston Marathon a record 61 times, running his last one in 1992 at the age of 84. After that, he continued on as the unofficial ambassador of the race, running part of it when he could. In those days, Johnny Kelley *was* the Boston Marathon. He came to represent the spirit of running—competitive when he could be, running as best he could later, and present as much as possible.

I was lucky enough to see him at the Boston Marathon in 1994, the first time I ran the race. He stood up on a stage at the runner's village before the race and serenaded the crowd with a version of "Young at Heart." It had become his theme song, and though his singing voice was nothing to write home about, the crowd clearly adored him, and he loved them back.

Johnny Kelley died in 2004 at the age of 97, just days before he was to go into a nursing home. That seemed fitting because I couldn't picture Johnny Kelley in such a place. He was a runner, and in my mind, he always would be. He's who I want to be when I grow up.

A THOUGHT EXPERIMENT

As we get older, we can look back on the phases of our lives as being like chapters, each with its distinctive theme. The Teenage Years, the College Experience, the First Job, and so on. Sometimes these chapters seem so distinct that we can feel disconnected from our memories of ourselves, almost as if we're thinking of someone that we used to know very, very well but with whom we've lost touch.

Imagine now that you've reconnected with one of these past selves and that you're both having a coffee in a café. You know all about them, of course, but they know nothing about you. So you tell them what you've been doing for the past decade or so.

What do you think their reaction will be? Admiration? Disappointment? Excitement and envy? Confusion? Will they like who you've become?

Since this is a book about running, we can focus for a moment on what you tell them about your training and racing. Perhaps they'll be surprised that you are a runner at all, or that it's become such an important part of your life. Perhaps they'll be surprised as well by your racing stories and accomplishments.

When you're done telling your past self everything you want to share, how do you feel? Proud of what you've done, or regretful?

The point of this exercise is to find an honest listener to share your history with, someone whom you trust to be honest with you, and whom you know that you can't lie to—yourself—to gain insight into how you feel about the choices you've made over the years. It's a moment to stop and take a deep breath and consider the path you've taken.

For most of us, our memories produce a mixed bag of feelings, stretching from pride and satisfaction to regret and disappointment. By focusing on our history in this way, we give ourselves the opportunity to be proud of what we've accomplished, with our running and in other things, while also highlighting ways in which we can learn from our past and make positive changes going forward. With some hard work and a little luck, the next time we share a coffee with a past self, we'll have even more good news to share.

ADJUST YOUR TRAINING

For me, the wonderful thing about running is figuring out what works. Our bodies are puzzles to be solved, and the fun comes from tinkering with all the factors within our control. But then, after we think we've figured out what works best for us, aging shakes up the whole game-board, forcing us to figure out new solutions to these problems.

Don't try to slap old answers onto these new problems; embrace the intellectual challenge and come up with new solutions. It will be a process of trial and error as you experiment with different distances, speeds, routines, and recovery periods, but eventually you'll nail it, and you'll become the kind of older runner you had hoped to be.

To continue to run and race as effectively as possible as we age, we need to adjust our routine. For those who haven't been doing strength and balance work earlier—and you should have been!—now is the time to get on track with it. Consider cross-training anew or taking fitness classes. Don't be afraid to experiment with new modes and methods of training.

Consider again how we can think of our bodies as being like friends of ours. At this point in our long relationship with our bodies, we need to give it extra care and attention. As one of my favorite spin and stretching instructors likes to say, treat your body like it belongs to someone you love. If you do, you'll find that while it might not be as spry as it was decades earlier, it can still pleasantly surprise you.

Further, being older doesn't mean that we can't be competitive athletes. We know that we will never again be fast enough to run with the young guns, but we don't have to. Our sport has created a category of competition just for us.

THE MASTERS RUNNER

The essence of a sports competition is for similarly gifted athletes to face one another on the field of battle, letting their skill and fitness determine who is the better athlete that day.

It would be no great victory for a much more gifted athlete to beat a lesser opponent. It would not be good for the athletes or for the sport. That's why boxing and bodybuilding have weight categories. And because an older runner is at a distinct physical disadvantage when trying to compete against much younger runners, the master runner category was invented.

A masters runner is simply any competitor who is over 40 years of age. Race directors usually further divide this category into 10-year increments, giving similar runners a chance to battle it out against each other as they age.

For many runners, aging into the masters category is at first a bitter pill to swallow, since it means that we have officially crossed over into our senior years. But any negativity usually evaporates when the benefits of being a masters runner become clear. Instead of being a mediocre (or worse) racer, masters runners can suddenly aim to qualify for racing in the Boston Marathon and vie for awards and even for prize money.

The philosophy behind the masters category is that a hard effort by a senior runner should be viewed in the context of their peer group, the way a hard effort by a younger athlete is ranked according to their finishing times in the open category.

Figuring out the best way to analyze relative effort levels led to the development of age-graded race calculators. These tools can tell you how your performance compares to the expected best times for runners in that age, gender, and race category. For example, a 65-year-old male masters runner could plug in his finishing time into the online calculator and see that his effort scored an 82 percent. He could then use this objective data to compare his times against all other runners in that race to see how he did overall.

The age-graded race calculator can be used not only across categories in a single race to judge your performance, but also against your younger self. In this way, I discovered that my finishing time in the Sydney Marathon one year as a masters runner was actually the best performance of my career, even though it was nine minutes slower than my overall personal record, set many years earlier. That's because my effort in Sydney was better, relative to other runners my age, than any of my earlier performances.

Thank you, Age-Graded Race Calculator!

CHAPTER NINE

THE FINISH LINE

"I run the marathon to make it beautiful."

—Uta Pippig,
Boston Marathon champion

Congratulations! You have reached the end of our journey. It's a path that took me decades to cover, but now you and I have made the trip in just a few hundred pages. We have achieved that rarest of all attributes: self-knowledge. Being a runner—*thinking* like a runner—means that we understand who we are and what we need to do to become our best selves. This is no small thing.

We've accomplished more than that, however. When we run, we do so not just for ourselves, but also as ambassadors of our sport. Whether we are aware of it or not, we all represent not just running but the entire running lifestyle and philosophy to our friends, our coworkers, our neighbors, and the world. When we run with joy, we encourage others to run, and in doing so, we enable them to come a bit closer to being their best selves as well.

But this isn't enough. Having reached this point, we have one more job to do, if we are willing to take it on. We need to give back. Just as no man is an island, no runner is a soloist. By now you know how much you've benefited from the encouragement and wisdom of others to become a runner. When you shopped for gear, went for group runs, raced, and read running blogs, magazines, and books (even this one), you were part of a community. That community thrives and serves us all when we all work to build it up. There are many ways to do so.

Join a running club. In most cities there are organized, nonprofit running clubs. The smallest ones might organize an annual Thanksgiving Day Turkey Trot and a weekly group run, and the largest, like the Boston Athletic Association and the New York Road Runners Club, produce huge marathons and a host of other races, as well as a wide range of classes, coaching opportunities, and other services. What they all do is connect people and strengthen the bonds that support our sport. Support them in turn if you can with your membership and your participation.

Support your local running shop. Running stores usually do so much more than sell gear and clothing; they are local centers for our sport. They support our community by offering group runs and race-targeted training, sometimes even producing their own races. Many are small family-owned, family-operated businesses. Consider spending your money there instead of at a big box store or online.

Volunteer. No race can exist without an army of volunteers. Every part of race production, from handing out race numbers, to placing trash bins, to manning aid stations, and so much more, requires the effort of unpaid workers. As a racer, I am acutely aware of how much I rely on all of them. Thank them as much as possible when you race, and consider volunteering when you're not racing.

Being a race volunteer is actually a fascinating job for a runner, especially if you volunteer at the finish line in a marathon. You can learn so much about the race experience. As a runner, all you see is the crowd around you, but as a volunteer, you witness the entire living, breathing animal that is a field of runners.

The first wave you'll see crossing the finish line is the elite runners, and they are truly otherworldly. Most of them hardly acknowledge you as they move through the finish line area, dealing with the race director and media.

The next wave is runners who are pressing hard to make their time goal. They suffer the most of all. Often these are the runners who collapse or vomit. Almost all of them are too wrapped up in their own suffering to acknowledge anyone else.

Next, finally, are the back-of-the-pack runners. These are people who simply had a dream of finishing. They are tired, but not suffering the way the faster runners did. And they *see* you. They'll thank you, and sometimes even hug you. They are the happiest of all runners.

I come away from these volunteering gigs thinking about what kind of runner I am, and if it's the kind of runner I want to be. On such days, volunteering has given me more than it's taken.

Sometimes, though, volunteering can provide unexpected moments. When working once at a big-time marathon expo, I asked a woman what her goal was for the race the next day. She told me that she wasn't actually running; she was there to support her boyfriend, who was competing. "But," she confided in me, "I've been told that I have the feet of a runner." I considered all the gnarled, calloused, black-nailed runner's feet I've seen over the years. "I'm not sure that was a compliment," I said.

Mentor. This is one of the sainted jobs in volunteering. While it's great to help with a race or support a run club, the best way to give back, in my own view, is to work with a young person and encourage them to run.

I've been lucky enough to work with some extraordinary people over the years who have created nonprofit organizations to encourage at-risk youth to get into running, and the experience has been amazing. Not just in the obvious ways, like getting to know the kids and helping them build up their fitness and health, but in the more subtle lessons that come with running, like learning about delayed gratification, patience, and persevering through adversity.

But there's something more. One of the groups I'd worked with partnered with a very big 10-mile race. High school kids would train with their mentors through the school year, with weekend group runs and separate mentor-student sessions, and then we would all gather on race day to compete.

These kids had trained for months and were ready, but they had little idea of what the race experience would be like until they showed up at the starting area. There they encountered thousands of other runners who shared their goal, and who would understand immediately how much work it took for them to get to that point.

The young runners realized then that they were not alone; that they were part of a community—the mythic big tent that encompasses people of all ages, faiths, ethnicities and backgrounds, gathered together for one purpose: to express ourselves through our running, and show ourselves and everyone else what we are all capable of.

Who wouldn't want to be a part of that?

Look for a group in your area that offers this kind of experience to kids, or better yet, start your own group. It will not just change their lives; it will change yours.

At the beginning of this book, we established that you are a runner when you decide that you are. Now we can add that you think like a runner when you become a runner who thinks about running. You now have the tools; go make this sport your own.

ACKNOWLEDGMENTS

Producing a book is always a team effort. My biggest thanks goes first to my wife, Stephanie Kay, who supported my move away from a legal career to fitness, and all my projects since. She's been my partner for so many adventures; hopefully there will be many more to come.

Thanks also to my son, Alex. Finding him waiting for me just past the finish line of my 200th marathon made that my best race ever.

I also owe thanks to my sisters Marlene Castricato and Dori Horowitz—they don't run, but they are Olympic-caliber supporters and cheerleaders.

Thanks as well to my editor Kierra Sondereker and the whole team at VeloPress; you make dreams come true!

Finally, a big thanks to all my clients, students, and teammates. A special thanks goes out to Frank Nasta, Marc Owens-Kurtz, and all my other running friends past and present. Together we are so much more than the sum of our parts. Run on!

ABOUT THE AUTHOR

Jeff Horowitz is a certified running, cycling, and triathlon coach and a personal trainer who has run more than 200 marathons and ultramarathons across six continents. Formerly an attorney, he quit law to pursue his passion for endurance sports. He currently teaches running at the George Washington University and works with runners aged 14 through 80. Horowitz is the author of *Quick Strength for Runners, Smart Marathon Training: How to Run Your Best Without Running Yourself Ragged, My First 100 Marathons: 2,620 Miles with an Obsessive Runner*, and *Ageless Strength: Strong and Fit for a Lifetime*.